Journey
^{to} Wellness

Journey
to Wellness

**Designing a People-Centred
Health System for Canadians**

Dr. R. Vaughan Glover

*Thank you for being part of this
forum!*

*All the best on your personal
journey.*

Vaughan

Jan 22/2010

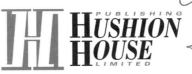
PUBLISHING
HUSHION
HOUSE
LIMITED

Library and Archives Canada Cataloguing in Publication

Glover, R. Vaughan, 1950-
    Journey to wellness : designing a people-centred health system for Canadians / R. Vaughan Glover ; illustrator, Bill Buttle.

"Taking back control of our health care—Only you can fix Canada's health care crisis".

ISBN 0-9733212-7-X

    1. Health care reform—Canada—Citizen participation.
2. Health promotion—Canada. 3. Medical policy—Canada—Citizen participation.

I. Title.

RA449.G56 2005   362.1'0971   C2005-904629-5

Book design by Fortunato Design Inc.
Cover design by Greg Rouble

Printed and bound in Canada

CONTENTS

INTRODUCTION

I invite you to join me as we explore together how our health system can put the health needs of each person first. It is an idea whose time has come.

IN OCTOBER 2003 I was honoured to win the top award for designing an American health system. It was an international competition sponsored by a group of concerned health leaders and citizens from Washington and Oregon. They were frustrated with their health system and the lack of vision and decided to challenge the grassroots to stimulate new ideas. They were overwhelmed with the response.

I had entered because a friend, Randy Atwater, had seen the announcement about the contest on a website and challenged me to enter. Randy and I had been discussing health reform and he had often given me feedback on my ideas to reform the Canadian health system.

Initially I was very hesitant about being associated with the American health system. Would people think I was trying to Americanize our beloved Canadian health system? My goal was to make a difference in Canada, and there is a real risk that many Canadians will not even listen to ideas if they have anything to do with the American way of thinking.

Randy's dare went something like this: "You have done all the work, so why not enter? You have nothing to lose and besides, if they recognize your ideas in the States, they may start to listen to you in Canada." How prophetic!

What I discovered is that although I am very proud of the accomplishments of our Canadian health system, neither country has discovered the perfect design. Perhaps we can learn from one another— if not what to do, at least what not to do.

We Need to Question the Status Quo and Be Active in Our Health

Of all the rights and freedoms we enjoy in Canada, the right to have choices in how we take care of ourselves is one that we seem to have taken for granted. Our right to become all we are capable of—to define our personal balance of mental, physical, spiritual and emotional well-being—is something we all assume exists. Unfortunately, without our even realizing it, that right is being eroded.

The American psychotherapist Dr. Wayne Dyer suggests that to make our desires come true you must, "change the way you look at things, and the things you look at will change."[1] Information is changing the way we look at things in life and society, and health care is no exception. Health care is moving toward a people-centred model that is based on listening, caring and trusting. It is high-quality care that is not judged solely on the ability to treat illness. It is relationship-based health care, founded on trust and respect and on accepting personal responsibility. Rewards are determined by how well the needs of the individual are met—not by how many people are treated but by how well each individual is treated. Informed Canadians appreciate the support our system offers, compared to many other countries, but we are beginning to see things differently. We are frustrated because we can't access this evolving level of care in our own country.

Frustration and resentment are mounting as the *Canada Health Act* has celebrated its 21st anniversary on April 1, 2005. Over the past two decades, change has happened in almost every aspect of health: who can deliver care, who should deliver care, what care can be delivered, people's values and goals for care, consumer knowledge and understanding, and the ability of the individual to be an active participant in his or her personal health. But through all of this, the Canada Health Act has remained the same.

...health and health care are unique to each individual and the public system must recognize and support all definitions of health.

We are beginning to realize that our current health system and the organizations that control and regulate it are resistant to change. They lack the political will to think outside the box. They either cannot or will not look at things from the perspective of the patient, nor appreciate that health and health care are unique to each individual and that the public system must recognize and support all definitions of health. The existing system is mired in bureaucracy, compromised by funding and management issues and unable to provide the excellence of care that we all want and deserve.

What Can We Do About It?

As the beneficiaries of an information age, Canadians have a responsibility and an opportunity to take a leadership role in the evolution of our health system. The change will be driven by an informed and empowered public, demanding access to what is possible rather than what a government or any other support group is willing or able to provide.

This book is about our *journey to wellness*, to an as yet undefined destination on our country's health continuum:

- enabling ordinary Canadians to make a difference and speed up the change from an "illness model" to a "wellness model" in which the patient is at the centre
- a health care model that uses teams of people supporting each patient in his or her goal to achieve a personally defined balance of mental, physical, spiritual and emotional health
- a health care model in which individuals regain ownership and control of their own health care
- embracing the reality that each individual is ultimately responsible for managing his or her own health and health care, and that the provider's role is to inform, empower and support rather than just fix and treat people, and
- acknowledging that we, the patients, must lead the way in building the next generation of health care in our country.

People-centred issues are very different from those usually raised by the media, health providers, politicians and health support groups. These special-interest groups are often concerned about issues like public vs. private, and for-profit or not-for-profit. Instead, the issues in

> *...the issues in a people-centred system are whether I feel valued, whether I am listened to, whether my needs are met, whether I was presented with all the options for care, and whether I received high-quality service.*

a people-centred system are whether I feel valued, whether I am listened to, whether my needs are met, whether I was presented with all the options for care, and whether I received high-quality service.

Thanks to the information age, the phrase "power to the people" is at last an achievable goal. Nowhere is this more needed than in health care, and nowhere is this more achievable than in Canada. As I will demonstrate throughout this book, Canada and Canadians are perfectly positioned to be world leaders in people-centred health reform. Health care is our number-one concern, and it is only right that we lead the way so others can follow. It is time for our Canadian voices to be heard.

My Personal Journey

I was raised in Marmora, a small mining town of 1,300 people in southern Ontario, the son of grocery-store owners and the grandchild of a minister. It was a caring and loving family who gave me the strong roots needed to pursue my own dreams.

Today, I am a 55-year-old dentist, and a happily married father of three. But that is just part of who I am. I am also a user of the health system, and it is from the perspective of a patient that I developed a people-centred proposal for health reform and wrote this book. I am a patient who has spent the past 30 years learning about myself, the people I work with, and the people I serve in my professional and personal life.

One of the most influential experiences in my teenage years occurred when I was 14, as a result of my habit of asking questions about everything. I had been reading an article in the *National Geographic* about the universe, infinity and where we came from, and it intrigued me. A short time later I had a lunch time discussion with some of my grade 10 classmates about heaven and hell and some of the biblical stories. I was questioning the physical existence of heaven and hell and upset some people. After all, it was 1964 and such talk was considered heresy. I was reported to the principal and sent home to discuss the matter with my parents, who then sent me off to talk to our minister, Rev. Maurice McLeod.

Reverend McLeod sat and listened quietly to my story, and his response has had an impact on me ever since. Instead of criticizing me and threatening me with the wrath of God for sinning, he said, "Vaughan, you just might be the luckiest person in our church. Our church, like all churches, is filled with people who have never asked those questions, either of themselves or others, and as a result they have never found the answers. They have faithfully come to worship and sat in the same pew and lived their whole lives with a faith based on what others tell them, not what they believe or have come to know." He explained that things of value in life don't often come easy and you have to challenge yourself and work to find the answers. He went on to say that if I kept asking those questions I would eventually find the answers and develop my faith.

...things of value in life don't often come easy and you have to challenge yourself and work to find the answers.

That was absolutely the last thing I expected to hear. He respected me, and instead of acting like a power figure he gave me responsibility and challenged me to deal with the issue. Instead of overpowering, he empowered.

Our health system is one of those things of great value in life, and as I have been researching for this book, I have often thought back to that time with Rev. McLeod. I cannot help but see the many politicians sitting in the front pews of the health hierarchy who have never asked the important questions about health, health care and a health system. Even more remarkable is that the people who are supposed to be the leaders and visionaries— prime ministers and premiers, federal and provincial ministers of health and deputy ministers—haven't asked the questions either, questions such as:

• Is there anything we agree on about health and health care?

- What is health? What is health care?
- Do we have an illness system or a health system? What does that mean, and what would a health system be like? How would it change our current model?
- Is the *Canada Health Act* actually a health insurance Act? What does that mean, and what would a health Act be like?
- Are the principles of the *Canada Health Act* actually insurance principles? What would health principles be, and how would we develop a system around health principles?
- Should health care be patient-centred, or is that just an election term? What would a working model be like if it were designed to inform and empower the individual as the manager of his or her personal well-being?
- What is wellness, and what would a well nation be like?
- How would you manage and fund a system that informs and empowers the individual?
- Do we want the people to be informed about their health and health care? How can we use the tools of this information age to empower the individual?

Journey to Wellness asks each of these questions and many more. It is time to put them all on the table and demand that the leaders challenge their blind faith in the current system. If we do not ask the questions and are not willing to search openly for answers, then we will never experience the reward of being empowered as the managers of our well-being.

People First—Leading The Way In Health Reform

In 1994 I was still asking questions and no one was providing answers, so I responded to a request from Ontario's provincial government for citizen input on a Health Policy Advisory Committee. I worked hard to put together some ideas on health policy, and eventually became chairman of the committee for eastern Ontario. I volunteered my time and used my own money for travelling to Ottawa and Toronto because I wanted to make a difference, rather than just complain. But after two years nothing seemed to be happening.

At that point a senior advisor to the Minister of Health took me aside and explained about the bureaucracy. She had read my letters and proposals and applauded my ideas, but she said, "Unless you can convince the voting public to support your ideas for the next election, you are wasting your time because getting elected is the first priority of any government." In other words,

> *...public policy rarely has a vision that extends past the next election— the greatest ideas in the world are worthless if you are not in power.*

public policy rarely has a vision that extends past the next election— the greatest ideas in the world are worthless if you are not in power. She then went on to explain that the key to change is to motivate the grass roots, and that politicians are rarely the visionaries. I have since learned that politicians and their policies react to what the people want, based on political correctness, public-opinion polls and what will win the next election. It was true then and the recent provincial and federal elections demonstrated that it is still true.

Instead of giving up, I decided to continue to try to make a difference. I left the committee and started to develop ideas about motivating the grass roots and encouraging people to change the way they look at things. Writing this book is another step on the journey.

It is an incredible challenge to try to influence health reform, but after 30 years' experience as a health care provider I have strong opinions on the issues affecting the current state of the health system in Canada. The most important, in my view, is that the system is not people-centred, and I am determined to be a catalyst and advocate for Canadians to change that.

The signs of unrest and the need for change are regular occurrences. Few demonstrations of unrest will have a greater impact than the Quebec supreme court decision in June 2005.

As we enter the 21st century, health care is a constant concern. The public health care system, once a source of national pride, has become the subject of frequent and sometimes bitter criticism... [I]t seems clear that a health care service that does not attain an acceptable level of quality of care cannot be regarded as a genuine health care service. Low quality services can threaten the lives of users.
—Supreme Court of Canada, *Chaoulli v. Quebec (Attorney General)*, 2005 SCC 35 (9 June 2005, paragraphs 2 and 50)

This all happened because one person had the courage to ask the question "why" and demand the answer. The answer made national news and will influence political debate.

Finally the door is wide open to review what many have said should never be touched. Our health system is flawed, must evolve to something better and each of us has a responsibility to be part of the discussion.

The goal is to empower the individual as an integral part of health reform, and to allow the reader's voice to be heard.

I invite you to join me as we explore together how we can make a new, people-centred model work for us in Canada.

ACKNOWLEDGEMENTS

AS ANYONE WHO HAS ATTEMPTED to write a book will tell you, it is an enormous task that consumes your life. Presenting a vision of health care makes it that much more difficult. Although it has been a very exhausting and at times an unnerving process, it has also become one of my greatest joys and accomplishments. It has given me a remarkable opportunity to make a difference and has grown far beyond what I believed was possible four years ago. The vision has evolved and the book has now become a means to an end. The evolution of our health system is a possible dream.

Realizing the goal would never have been possible without the support of many very special people. I want to name a few and say thank you: Randy Atwater, who sat and talked for many hours and challenged me to go for it. The sisters at Still Point for the perfect environment for writing. Hon. Senator Marjory LeBreton, who was the first politician to take the time to listen. My mentors Dr. Duncan Sinclair, Doug Angus, Gilles Paquet and Dr. Bruce Squires, who took the time to meet with a man from Arnprior with a vision and who have become major sources of inspiration and support. Ian Outerbridge, who has been a marvellous support and spent countless hours on the phone helping me to stay in control of all that is happening. Marion Balla, who has played a major role in all that I have learned and challenged me to become all I am capable of. Dr. Harold Worth, Dr. L.D. Pankey and everyone at the Pankey Institute who were instrumental in starting me on my journey to relationship-based health care. Kathleen O'Connor and the visionaries at *Code Blue Now!*, for creating the opportunity for the grassroots to have their messages heard. Meghan Cross, who edited my presentation to Design an American Health System. Serena Williamson, who did the initial edits on the book. Bill Tatham, Errol Singer and the whole team at XJ Partners who have been a wonderful support and have opened up so many doors.

To all the clients in our practise whom I have had the pleasure to serve and learn from, thank you.

To Dr. Bruce Nesbitt, who has patiently worked with me for many months to edit the final product and has given me the confidence to continue, I say thank you.

To Bill Buttle for his wit, humour and insightful cartoons, that help us all to lighten up and change the way we look at things. I say thank you.

To my whole people-centred office team, who are like family, who have been an integral part of this incredible journey and who are the working model on which much of this vision is based, I say thank you.

To my partners, Tony and Christina, thank you for your patience and support.

To mom, dad and all my family who have given me love and support through all the years, thank you.

Finally, to Betsy, Amy, Chris and Laura, this book is dedicated to you. It is the love of family and friends that pushes each of us to make a difference. Thank you for your patience.

PART I

What Needs to Be Done

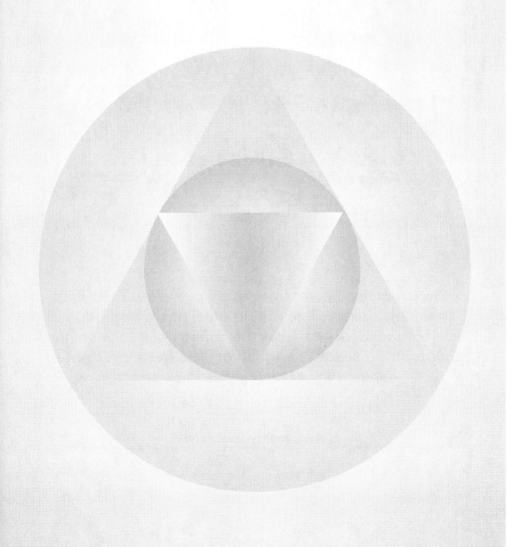

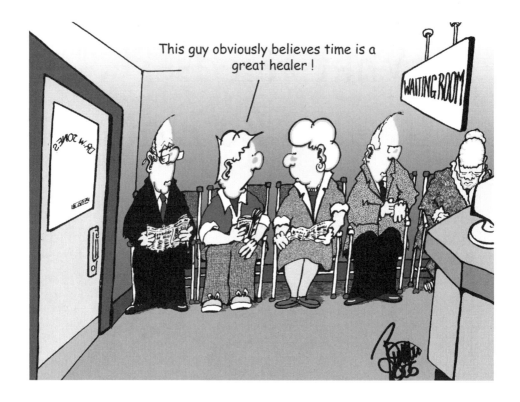

*"Governments have promised on numerous occasions
to find a solution to the problem of waiting lists.
Given the tendency to focus the debate on a sociopolitical
philosophy, it seems that governments have lost sight of
the urgency of taking concrete action."*

C *Supreme Court of Canada*, Chaoulli v. Quebec
(Attorney General), *2005 SCC 35*
(9 June 2005, paragraph 96)

CHAPTER 1

What Went Wrong with Canada's Health Care System?

Health care is now a $130 billion a year business and there is still no vision, no plan and no coherent policy.

O NE OF THE THINGS I value most in life is to be able to dream, to have a vision and pursue it, to become all I am capable of by design and not by accident. Similarly health care and the health system must support a dream or vision for health that is relevant to the needs and expectations of individual Canadians.

After years as a provider studying the existing health system and witnessing its effect on the lives of Canadians, I find that the current system is both a positive and a negative influence on my ability to conceive and achieve my vision.

On the positive side, one of the most important accomplishments of our country in the past 50 years is that Canadians made a commitment as a nation to support the health of the people. This sets us apart from many nations and is still the number one concern of most people. It is a wonderful support to have access to a universally defined level of care. But as our health goal moves from treating illness to supporting a much broader definition of health, the same system can be one of the greatest barriers to fulfilling health dreams because it places all kinds of conditions and rules on both the provider and the patient.

Most people have never analyzed the impact of the current health system. Twenty years ago it was considered a model for the world; our politicians still tell us it is one of the best in the world, and we celebrate it without questioning. The reality is that the best in the world

20 years ago is not necessarily the best in the world today. Headlines like "Mediocre Care at High Price" and "Canada Ranked 15th for MRIs and 14th for Life Expectancy" only stir the fires of unrest.[2]

The Origins and Aims of Today's Medicare

Universal health insurance for Canadians was instituted by the national *Medical Care Act* of 1966, largely sparked by Premier Tommy Douglas' introduction of medicare in Saskatchewan four years earlier. Douglas came to be considered the father of medicare, and through his work and that of many other politicians and visionaries, eventually Canada developed the five principles on which the present Canadian system is founded. They were updated in 1984 when the current *Canada Health Act* was passed but remain essentially the same.[3]

Today, the five basic principles of the *Canada Health Act* form the foundation for health care in Canada:

- *comprehensiveness*: all medically necessary services inside or outside hospitals must be covered by the provinces
- *accessibility*: services must be reasonably accessible anywhere in Canada
- *universality*: all Canadians must have coverage for the medically necessary services defined under the plan
- *public administration*: health insurance for what are defined as medically necessary hospital and doctor services must be managed and paid for through public funding, and any alternative funding must be universal, and
- *portability*: the services must be portable from province to province.

When I first started to study medicare, Douglas' vision in the 1960s was related to me this way. In a country as affluent as Canada there are two objectives:

1. We cannot tolerate that all people do not have a universal level of care for emergencies, life-threatening illnesses, accidents and treatable illness and disease.

2. We cannot tolerate that people will go bankrupt attempting to provide the basic health care needs for themselves or their loved ones.

The *Canada Health Act* and the five principles are a credit to the commitment of Canadians to ensure that all citizens have access to high-quality health care without fear of a crippling financial burden. Although we can always improve, we have addressed these two goals and everyone has access to basic illness and emergency care.

The problem is that the vision is nearly 40 years old, and we are now aiming too low.

But health is like all things in life—once you reach one goal, there is always another. The problem is not that we have failed to achieve our goals; the problem is that there is so much more to health in 2005 than the leaders and visionaries ever imagined in 1966 or even in 1984. The problem is compounded as people become informed about what is possible and they demand access to all options. The problem is that the vision is nearly 40 years old, and we are now aiming too low.

The Four Pillars of Health Care

As I researched the literature from a patient's perspective, I discovered there are four pillars of support for all health systems.

- The central pillar is the *individual* with the health problem: the patient, client, consumer or user of the health system. These are the people for whom the system is intended. The individual defines and represents health.
- The second pillar is the *provider*: the doctor, nurse, chiropractor, health team, clergy or therapist—any individual group or organization that supports the well-being of each person needing care. When a provider fulfills a central role with the individual, he or she represents health care.
- The third pillar is the *support groups*: governments, drug companies, insurance companies, churches, health charities and so on. They include any individual, group or organization that

supports the well-being of the people or supports the primary provider or coach. These groups represent health support.

- The fourth pillar is the *system*: legislation, principles, definitions—anything that defines, manages or gives direction and sets boundaries for the other pillars. Collectively they represent the health system.

Each pillar exists in any health system, but what differentiates a patient-centred system from doctor-centred, politically-centred or insurance-centred systems is the role each of the pillars plays.

The Crumbling Four Pillars

1. *The individual*

After reviewing my proposed reasons to reform the health system, an Ottawa newspaper reporter went on to comment that "a group of politicians decides how much money health care is entitled to; another regime decides how much doctors will make and how many hospitals we can have. Another group decides—because resources are limited—what expensive tests will be available to whom. At the end of the food chain, in walks the patient, getting whatever care the system can eke out. If he needs to wait a year for a hip replacement so be it. The care is universal, it's accessible, it's affordable; it just isn't very good".[4]

Canadians are thankful for the level of support that we receive, but there is a growing feeling that we are not in control of our health support—that we are at the end of the food chain, rather than at the top where the politicians and the system said we should be.

When medicare was first introduced in Canada, it fulfilled the expectations and needs of the people. As time passed and expectations grew and changed, the inability of our system to keep pace with change became more obvious. And as the system's resistance to change and new ideas has become clear to the public, the inability of patients to be active change agents in improving the system leaves them feeling like helpless onlookers, waiting to see what is in it for them.

I have encountered many real life stories about the frustrations for the patient in the current system. Crystal, for example, is a long-time friend and client who called me at work in January 2004. She was in tears and asked if I could help since she knew I was trying to improve the system. Crystal had been having problems with her hip for some time, but in the previous two months her symptoms had developed into excruciating pain, regularly bringing her to tears. Her family doctor arranged an appointment with an orthopaedic surgeon who diagnosed a severe degenerative disorder, told her that she needed an immediate hip replacement and classified it as urgent. The problem for both Crystal and her doctor was that she must live with the pain and crippling symptoms for another year, simply because that was the earliest she could be treated.

This feeling of helplessness exists today, but information can be the factor that will change this. Information through books like this, journals, newspapers, the Internet, TV and radio is empowering Canadians with the confidence to have a voice in the design of a system that puts the health of the people at the head of the food chain.

Until now, the problem has been how to have your voice heard. I too was frustrated because there was no way to be heard, but discovered that the informed person can be the most powerful voice in the system. Since my ideas were recognized, the leaders of the movement to maintain the status quo don't know what to do with me. They can't fire me, because I am just a patient; they can't destroy my election campaign, because I am not running for election; and they can't accuse me of serving my own interests, because I don't work for the system and have funded all my years of work and research out of my own pocket.

In writing this book and founding the Canadian Association for People-Centred Health, I am an advocate for the patient, with the goal of finding a way to support the health of the people better. My personal mission is *to be an advocate for the people as a visionary and an architect for a people-centred health system.* I want to build a system around health, rather than asking people and providers to compromise their expectations and goals to fit a system.

> **My personal mission is to be an advocate for the people as a visionary and an architect for a people-centred health system.**

2. *The providers*

The providers—the coaches, doctors, nurses and health teams who provide the care—find themselves with better equipment, facilities and supportive techniques to treat illness and disease than they have ever had before. In addition, there is a universal health safety net that provides an acceptable level of support for basic care. The problem is that this level of care is managed by a bureaucracy that resists change and limits the services provided, even as the expectations and needs of the health consumer and provider are changing and expanding.

Providers are frustrated because they can celebrate what they are able to offer their clients, yet they realize that there is so much more that can be done. The current system is simply unable to keep pace.

Winning elections, effective lobbying by special interest groups, philosophical debates over profit vs. not-for-profit and public vs. private, powerful public-opinion polls: all have supplanted the evolving vision of care.

Information is constantly challenging providers with new research and techniques, but like their patients they feel as if they are passive observers helplessly watching and waiting to see when, where and how they can make use of the new technologies. They have lost much of their ability to fulfill the obligations of the Hippocratic oath sworn by most doctors—to serve the needs of the patient above all—not because they don't want to, but because patients' expectations and needs are moving beyond what the system is able to support and the system is creating barriers to any alternatives. Winning elections, effective lobbying by special interest groups, philosophical debates over profit vs. not-for-profit and public vs. private, powerful public-opinion polls: all have supplanted the evolving vision of care.

Yet there is an answer. Information is also empowering some providers to speak up and be heard. They are becoming visionaries in the design of a form of health care that supports the health needs of the people by whatever means possible. From the membership of the Ontario Medical Association refusing to accept a contract from the

Ontario provincial government to a medical doctor in Montreal willing to go to court to fight for his patients' right to care in a timely fashion, providers are beginning to refuse to accept policies that affect their relationships with their clients and the health of the people.[5]

3. *The support groups*

Whether it is federal or provincial politicians or pharmaceutical and insurance companies, support groups are increasingly frustrated with the lack of vision and clear policy in the current system.

The various *political support groups* have different missions and goals, but the common political goal is to implement a politically correct system based on public-opinion polls in which all people's needs are equal and are treated equally. After 40 years of a purportedly universal system, experience and research are showing that people are unique, not only in their needs but also in their wants and their values.

I challenge all Canadians to take the time to discuss health care with politicians, on a personal level, without media present. You will discover (as I have) that most politicians are confused and frustrated because, despite their efforts to be all things to all people, the people are not happy. Their attempts to impose universal solutions are too often failing to fulfill the unique health needs of the people. Informed people know there are options, and they want to have the choice of accessing what is possible rather than what a government or any third party is willing or able to offer, so the frustration grows.

Special-interest support groups (drug and insurance companies, for example) are equally frustrated. When I discussed a people-centred health reform model with the chief executive officer of a large pharmaceutical firm, he explained that on a personal level, everyone who works for these corporations is a patient of the same system, and their philosophy is to support the health of the people. Their ultimate corporate goal is to make a difference in the quality of life of their clients and to be rewarded appropriately. For years, profits were the first priority, but the media and an informed public are challenging health industries every day to put people first. These companies have the

potential to be great allies of a people-centred system, but clear public policy with a long-term vision must lead the way.

4. *The system*

Over 20 years have passed since the *Canada Health Act* was implemented in 1984, and virtually everything about health, health care and
health support has changed while the system has not.

The *Canada Health Act* seems to be untouchable, at least from a
political standpoint. Although the 1974 Lalonde Report focused on
prevention and health promotion, its recommendations have not
been reflected in governments' policy intentions.[6] The system is helplessly mired in partisan politics and autocratic legislation and guidelines that were designed to treat emergencies and illness. Patients and
their families are beginning to accept that it is impossible for a government to provide all options for care, but informed people also understand that governments are only one of many support options. If a
level of care is possible and a government or legislation is preventing
or delaying access because they can't afford it, then we can become
very cynical and bitter.

Health support beyond disease care is not achievable by a paternalistic model that does things *to* people. We accepted a paternalistic
model 40 years ago, but 40 years ago there were fewer options—and
more importantly, people did not have the information to know the
options. Health care today requires a system that empowers individuals to take responsibility and control, and empowers the support
groups to work with them.

So the system is struggling as well, trying to fulfill the political priority of getting the politicians re-elected and, at the same time, to support the ever-changing health needs of the people.

But there is a way out. Informed stakeholders will show the way by
putting their creative minds together to design principles, definitions
and legislation that will provide the boundaries and guidelines for the
next generation's health system—one that is patient-centred, supports
the health and well-being of each Canadian, and continues to provide
a health safety net we can all be proud of. This is our challenge.

The *But* Factor for Stakeholders

Perhaps the best way to summarize the dilemma for all stakeholders in the current system is that they are ultimately controlled by the *but* factor. Most health stakeholders (political or corporate) say they believe in informing and empowering the patient; this claim, however, is usually qualified by a *but*, such as: *but* only if it supports the most recent public-opinion poll or shareholder group. The *but* is often an absolute, non-negotiable qualifier. The political rhetoric of the 2004 federal election is an example: all the major political parties claimed their first priority was the health of the people, *but* all agreed that policies must be universal or not for profit. In other words, they actually believe in a not-for-profit or universal system, and the patient can only be informed and empowered to the extent that it fits into the system.

> There is a tremendous difference between a system-centred and patient-centred vision for health care. It is time to make the people's health the non-negotiable base.

In a people-centred system it is the other way around. The non-negotiable base is the health needs of the individual. For example, there should be a universal level of care *but* the individual ultimately must have the right to decide what level of care best meets his or her needs.

There is a tremendous difference between a system-centred and patient-centred vision for health care. It is time to make the individual's health the non-negotiable base.

The 85% Hip: How the Current System Works

There are many classic examples of how our current system fails to put the patient first. One is a story that an orthopaedic surgeon told me in 2002 highlighting one aspect of the conflict for doctors and the unknown risk for the patient.

We were discussing how decisions were made in the system. He said, "This year we are using the 85% hip." Needless to say I wanted to hear more, so he explained. Each year the Ontario provincial government decides what our budget will be for artificial hips. The surgeons then meet and evaluate all the hips on the market and this year they decided to use the 85% hip. This means that in the opinion of the surgeons, there were five or six acceptable hips on the market that ranged upward from the cheapest, which was 75% of the cost of the most expensive. The surgeons were faced with long waiting lists (up to two years for a so-called non-urgent hip replacement) and were forced to make a decision about which hip they would use, since it is not acceptable to give one person a certain quality of hip and another a different one. They decided that if they used the 85% hip, then they would be able to budget for 30 more hip replacements that year.

I then asked whether I could have the more expensive hip if it met my lifestyle better, or if I just plain wanted it. He explained that under the criteria, the most expensive ceramic hip was only for people under a certain age. So I asked if this meant a 40-year-old couch potato could get a ceramic hip, but the 55-year-old marathoner cannot. He confirmed that that is how the system works in the city of Ottawa. People assume they are getting the best because they trust their doctors. But it is not common practice to inform patients what the options are, because in the current system in Ontario there are no options. If everyone can't have it, then no one can have it.

My doctor friend went on to explain that this manner of determining health procedures is common throughout the system, whether it is for an examination, drug prescriptions, counselling or hospital equipment. The government determines the funding and the providers make the care fit the funding. The treatment options that are offered are based on what fits the system or what the government can finance, rather than what is possible or best for the individual patient. The legislation and the bureaucracy say that the principle of universality must come before the needs of any one patient.

This is how the system works. At the top are the federal, provincial and territorial governments. They collect the money and ultimately decide how many people with hip problems will be treated. Next are the doctors. They have some say, but are forced to compromise in an effort to serve the most people for the fewest dollars. They cannot use the facilities to their full extent because of budgets and rules. At the bottom are the Crystals in our society. Each of us knows someone who is experiencing a feeling of helplessness that is repeated every day for thousands of providers and patients, most without even understanding what is happening or why. The providers are not happy in the existing system, but they are unable or unwilling to bring about change.

As Canadians begin to ask questions they will realize there are choices and compromises made every day— without the patient ever knowing the difference— and too many of these choices affect the quality and even the length of someone's life.

The 85% hip is only one example. As Canadians begin to ask questions they will realize there are choices and compromises made every day—without the patient ever knowing the difference—and too many of these choices affect the quality and even the length of someone's life.

This does not mean that more expensive is better, but it should be the patient and his or her provider who make the decision, not the insurance company. It is time to change the way you look at things and ask the questions that need to be asked about your health, health care, health support and the health system.

The Question of Informed Consent

The legal and ethical issue of informed consent is raised by the fact that people receive 85% hips or 85% health care in any form to fit the financial realities of an insurance plan. In Canadian law, it is assumed that each patient has a right to give informed consent to treatment. This means that people have the right to know their options for health care, and providers have the obligation to inform their patients about the options before they provide treatment. When people begin to understand that there are always options and that it is impossible for any health support system—even our so-called universal system—to cover all options, and if the system continues to restrict options to what is covered, then there is a growing question about whether the right to informed consent is respected in the current system.

The dilemma for the provider is whether to support the universal principle and only offer what is covered by the universal plan, or to offer all options even if they are not covered. If you study the existing system and the way the average general practitioner works, you will begin to realize that it is the financial limitations of the system that are dictating the limitations of the care and the options presented, and that too often options are not given. Of course there are exceptions, and I am not suggesting that doctors do not try to inform before they perform, but the frustration with a system that is focused on insurance principles, not health principles, is creating a serious legal and ethical problem.

The problem for doctors is compounded because if they offer an option such as a 100% hip and the system only covers an 85% hip, then it is illegal for the patient to pay for the difference, and the doctor can be fined for accepting payment.[7] The doctor only has two choices: do it for nothing or don't offer the option. The fact that no doctor offers a 100% hip or for that matter a less expensive 75% hip where it is appropriate means that most have opted for the latter.

This ethical dilemma is another reason why doctors are frustrated, and some to the point that they decide to leave the country. An Ottawa doctor described as one of Canada's top cancer specialists moved to Houston, Texas in 2002. When asked why, he responded "rather than stay here, frustrated because I am not able to offer what I think is the highest quality of care and not being able to do what I consider the highest quality research, I think I have to go to Houston."[8] Perhaps all patients should be asking how often the current system puts doctors in a position where there is no option to violating the laws regarding informed consent.

The Critical Problem of Funding

The *Canada Health Act* commits the provincial and federal governments to provide insurance that is universal, comprehensive, accessible, portable, and publicly funded. To achieve this goal, both levels of government collect taxes—although the *Constitution Act, 1867* assigns primary responsibility for health care to the provinces—and then distribute the tax revenue for health care.

In 2004 the provincial governments invested $83.4 billion in health and the federal government spent $4.7 billion directly. The provincial and federal ministries of health are responsible for distributing these funds in such a way that they support the principles of the Act. (In addition, municipal governments spent $1 billion, social security funds distributed $1.8 billion, and the private sector spent $39.2 billion, for a national total of $130.2 billion.)[9]

The current Act prohibits a provider from accepting any form of remuneration for a procedure that is covered under the comprehensive clause of the Act. This means that the doctors are accountable to a public insurance company for their income, and the patient's opinion on the care and service is not really a part of the process.

Perhaps the greatest threat to our health care system is the financial inability of the governments to provide the comprehensive and timely universal level of care that an informed public defines as high-quality care. The risk of crisis rises as the expectations of informed patients continue to grow, while the financial capacity of the various levels of government is decreasing. These issues are highlighted in a commentary from the C.D. Howe Institute, *What Happened to Health-Care Reform?* (2003). The paper suggests that "provincial politicians should not pretend that simply adding more federal money will provide a lasting solution to the fiscal problems of the health system…. [N]otwithstanding the political rhetoric, it is not possible to 'buy' reform."[10]

The National Debt is Eroding Our Options

The massive federal, provincial and municipal debt that has accumulated over the past 30 years is now taking its toll on all social programs. The Canadian Institute for Health Information reported that in 2004, Canadian governments invested approximately $2,900 per person in health care through federal and provincial tax dollars.[11] At the same time, all levels of government spent an estimated $1,228 per person on interest on the combined debt, or about 43% of what we spend on health care—and all this when interest rates are at the lowest point in decades.[12]

As informed people begin to realize that our health care will be seriously compromised when there is an economic downturn (and there will be a downturn) with increased interest rates, they will want a system that can cope with economic change and give people alternatives.

Even if We Have the Resources We Can't Afford to Pay for Them

The system's inability to provide timely care is a serious concern, but informed Canadians are starting to understand that this is primarily a financial or system problem. There are operating rooms, artificial hips and knees, and surgeons to do the surgery, but the system is unable to fund the care that is required.

An expert panel concluded in 2001 that "by 2010, even with focused efforts to manage demand, encourage comprehensive practise and make more effective use of other health care providers, Ontario will need over 1,300 new physicians."[13] Financially, even if 1,300 new physicians arrived tomorrow, the system could not afford to employ them.

The shortage of diagnostic equipment such as MRIs and computerized axial tomography (CT) scans is seriously affecting the quality and timeliness of care. According to a recent study by the Fraser Institute, Canada is ranked 15th out of 24 Organization for Economic Co-Operation and Development (OECD) countries and 17th out of 23 for CT scan availability.[14] To accentuate the serious nature of the financial crisis, even if there were more units the government could not afford to operate them.

Many MRI and CT units sit idle for hours each day because there is inadequate funding.[15] It makes no sense to invest in more units if we can't afford to use the units we already have efficiently and effectively. To make matters even worse, not only are the units used inefficiently but the ones we have are outdated and incapable of giving the diagnostic information that more technologically advanced units are able to provide. If the government can't provide a service well, it has two options: either it should openly declare what support it is able to offer given the shortcomings and allow people to pursue other choices, or it should get out of the business.

The shortages of nurses, nurse practitioners, specialists and hospital beds are all serious concerns. The Canadian Nurses Association estimated that there were only 993 nurse practitioners in Canada in 2003.[16] Effectively using nurse practitioners could help relieve the doctor shortage, but the system does not encourage expanded use of alternative providers and one reason is that it cannot afford to employ them.

Each of these examples (and many more) highlight a system that is strained to the limit to provide the status quo, and yet is not close to providing the quality and timeliness of care that we know is possible. The publicly funded support system just can't afford the service we want.

...highlight a system that is strained to the limit to provide the status quo, and yet is not close to providing the quality and timeliness of care that we know is possible.

The System Has Lost Sight of The Patient

With all the debate about the Canadian health care system and its importance to us as a country and a society, we have somehow lost sight of the patient. It is on this realization that all my efforts are founded.

There are books about political solutions to political problems, health care delivery and the crisis for nurses, doctors and all other providers; and books about the need for stronger controls and the need to save what some people believe is one-tiered health care. Most recently, Canadians have invested millions of dollars in the Kirby and Romanow studies on health care reform.[17] It is interesting to note that even though there are many references in the literature to making health care patient-centred, not one book or study has focused on the patient as the centre.

Instead, our Canadian health care system is focused on professional and political agendas fullfilling the principles of the health act — a one-tiered philosophy — and not on the health of the individual. Consider:

- The median wait time for knee replacements in Ontario was 33 weeks during 2003–2004 (that is, half of the patients waited longer), and for cancer surgery (radical prostatectomy) it was nearly three months.[18]

- Growth and options are limited by the publicly funded health care system because health care priorities are determined by political agendas and public-opinion polls. Priorities in the provision of health care are often based on getting politicians re-elected. The system is politically focused, not people-focused.
- Our governments are going bankrupt and compromising other social programs trying to meet the health expectations of the public, and would probably be bankrupt if they had sufficient nurses, doctors, support staff and equipment to service the needs of the people without unreasonable waiting lists.
- The universal average care on which the system is built is rarely the same as individual excellence.
- Providers are frustrated because of a lack of control and the need to adhere to the limitations of the system.
- The system is resistant to change. In Canada it is political suicide for a government even to put an alternative model on the table for discussion. Patients, providers and support are changing, but our collective belief that the Canadian system is the best and shouldn't be changed remains steadfast.
- There is no reward for providing high-quality care. It is against the law for a health care provider to be rewarded for providing a service beyond the government's accepted norm. As an example, a doctor receives the same fee for delivering a baby whether the patient has fifteen minutes or fifteen hours of labour. Providers can be fined for billing for higher-quality services than the average recognized in the universal system.
- Waiting lists have become a tool for governments to defer payment for treatment. Many patients must either leave the province or even the country or break the law to get a service when they want or need it. Politicians indirectly dictate when services will be delivered. (Coincidentally, Crystal was in so much pain that she could not tolerate the Ontario waiting lists, so she went to Quebec and paid to have her hip replaced in less than two weeks)

Canadians must ask why we are willing to compromise the health of the people to fit a 40-year-old system, while it is almost considered treason to explore options for creating a system that can adapt to the health needs of the people.

Perverse Incentives

Despite all the time, energy, financial resources and political will that have been devoted to creating a functional Canadian health system, we still find ourselves in a country where counterproductive requirements are built into that system. In his book *Code Blue* (1999), Dr. David Gratzer compiled a "cynic's list of perverse incentives" that outlines the scope of the problem that is confronting Canadians, and highlights many of the reasons why Canadians must continue to search for ways to save their beloved health system.[19]

It's interesting that each of his perverse incentives is related to one of four things:

- the financial crisis
- health care providers and supporters not being accountable to the patient
- the patient not being responsible for treatment or reward, or
- the challenge of simultaneously winning an election and managing a health system.

Here is a shortened version of Dr Gratzer's list of perverse incentives. No doubt you will recognize many of them from your own experience.

Incentives for the patient

- Patients have an incentive to use the emergency room as a 24-hour office of a family physician. Emergency rooms are convenient.
- Patients have an incentive to run to the walk-in clinic for every minor ailment, including the common cold. Walk-in clinics are easily accessible, and the consultation is fast.
- Patients have an incentive to get every diagnostic test for even

the most minor complaints. Tests provide peace of mind and
they are free.

- Patients have an incentive to have every ache and pain of old
age checked out. Aches and pains of old age require no treatment, but attention is nice.

Incentives for the doctor

- Doctors have an incentive to order many tests. Tests make the
diagnoses easier and keep patients happy.
- Doctors have an incentive not to treat complicated cases.
Complicated cases are rarely compensated adequately.
- Doctors have an incentive to see healthy patients frequently.
Visits from healthy patients make for healthy incomes.
- Doctors have an incentive to treat minor illnesses. Minor
illnesses are easy to treat, and they pay well.

Incentives for the health care administrator

- Health care administrators have an incentive to introduce
new, redundant services. Expansion increases global budgets.
- Health care administrators have an incentive to negotiate rigid
contracts with unions representing orderlies, food workers,
and other support staff. Contractual limitations help to
enlarge global budgets.
- Health care administrators have an incentive not to contract
services out. Fewer services require fewer administrators.
- Health care administrators have an incentive to limit government
restructuring efforts. Restructuring kills administrative jobs.

Incentives for the politicians

- Politicians have an incentive not to close redundant hospitals.
Closures are politically unpopular.
- Politicians have an incentive not to clash with health care
administrators, unions and doctors. Disagreements make poor
public spectacles.

- Politicians have an incentive not to change the system. Medicare is popular.
- Politicians have an incentive to make cost-cutting decisions for short-term budgetary gain that result in higher costs in the long term. Short-term gains reflect the short-term reality that the next election is always just around the corner.
- Politicians have an incentive to allow waiting lists to develop. Some type of cost control must occur.
- Politicians have an incentive not to invest in high-tech diagnostic equipment. MRI and CT scanners are expensive to buy and run.
- Politicians have an incentive to limit a doctor's ability to practise medicine. The doctor–patient relationship is important, but saving money is more important.
- Politicians have an incentive to allocate resources to service the government's voter base better. Politicized medicine has political results.

We must ask ourselves why, after investing millions of dollars in studies and soliciting solutions from some of the best minds in the world, we have a system where each of these perverse incentives is alive and well.

The *Canada Health Act* Is Not a Health Act

As proud as I am that our country is committed to a universal level of health support, there are serious shortcomings with the way the system has evolved or failed to evolve. The *Canada Health Act* was only the beginning. The problems I have discussed so far demonstrate that the Act and the way it is implemented must change.

As I researched and wrote about our health system, it became obvious that the apparently untouchable *Canada Health Act* is actually an insurance act, or worse still, a political act. For the past ten years I have been saying this, but until recently, very few leaders publicly agreed with this fact. Now that information in the media is beginning to expose the real facts, it seems that many people are beginning to admit it is a health-financing or insurance act, at best. Even Monique

Bégin, the Minister of National Health and Welfare who brought in the *Canada Health Act* in 1984, now refers to it as our "universal health insurance system" and suggests that it should be de-politicized.[20]

This means that the piece of legislation guiding our health system is not a health Act that defines health and what we are supporting: it is a health insurance Act that defines how the government will support this as yet undefined entity called health. The five principles of the *Canada Health Act* are not so much principles of health as they are the principles that any insurance company sets out for a client in an insurance policy. *Universality* is whom they cover. *Comprehensive* is a statement about what they will cover. *Accessibility* is where you can receive coverage. *Portability* means that your insurance covers you regardless of what province you are in. *Public funding* defines who is paying the premiums.

> *What is missing is a clear understanding of the difference between insurance principles and health principles*

What is missing is a clear understanding of the difference between insurance principles and health principles (discussed in Chapter 3). As we move to the next generation of our health system, it is essential that we actually create a health Act and health principles that will clearly define what the insurance Act is supporting. Then we can rename the current Act to take its proper place as a guide for financial support.

We Need a Vision—For The People, By The People

There are several things about the status quo that most Canadians want to keep:

- a high-quality universal level of emergency and disease care that is available to all Canadians regardless of financial or social status
- a funding mechanism to support this level of care, and
- assurance that no Canadian goes bankrupt trying to obtain basic health care.

But the four pillars of Canada's health system *(page 6)* are eroding.

Each of the participants has different goals, objectives and problems. There is no vision or common mission that binds them all.

This realization is not new. It is just that no one has done anything about it. As Michael Rachlis and Carol Kushner noted in *Second Opinion* (1989), "perhaps the most astounding discovery anyone studying our health care system will make is that it operates without any overall objectives at all. There is no plan, no vision, no coherent policy. We're running a $46 billion operation with no idea of what we're trying to achieve. Can you imagine any other industry of that size neglecting such a fundamental imperative?"[21] The most unbelievable part is that 15 years later, the business is now a $130 billion operation and there is still no vision, no plan and no coherent policy.

If the health leaders won't put forward a vision for health and health care then the leadership must come from the people. This book challenges each of us to do our part.

It seems incredible, but for 20 years Canadians have been debating and politicians have lost and won elections over the health care system, and yet no one has ever clarified what the system is supporting and what it is ultimately supposed to do. Is the purpose of the system to treat illness or to support a much broader definition of health? Is it to support a political philosophy or a business portfolio or the shareholders of a major corporation? Is it to support a particular ideology on funding health care or is it to support the health of the people by whatever means are available?

It seems incredible, but for 20 years Canadians have been debating and politicians have lost and won elections over the health care system, and yet no one has ever clarified what the system is supporting and what it is ultimately supposed to do.

None of these questions has been answered. In fact, we cannot even agree on a definition of health. It is essential for us to institute a health Act that clearly defines health for today and the future. Once we decide what "health" means, then we can start to develop the principles of a real people-centred health system. That is where the next two chapters will take us.

SUMMARY—CHAPTER 1

When we assess the problems in our current health system, we should:

- celebrate the fact that we live in a country that is committed to supporting the health of its people, but accept that everything about health and health care is changing and the system must evolve

- recognize that the challenge is to have the patient come first, not the system

- decide whether 85% health care is acceptable, so long as the options are clear and the choice is made by the person receiving the care

- question whether informed consent is a fundamental right that must be respected

- accept that inadequate funding and debt servicing are realities that force us to change the way we look at things

- understand that the perverse incentives of a 40-year-old vision are destroying the system

- acknowledge that the *Canada Health Act* is an insurance act, not a health act

- challenge ourselves and others to create a vision that can evolve with the expectations of an increasingly informed and empowered population, and

- have the courage to ask the questions and the commitment to find the answers that will help us to be world leaders in health care once again.

CHAPTER 2

A New Definition of Health

Health is a personally defined balance of mental, physical, spiritual and emotional well-being.

THE FIRST STEP on our journey to wellness is to identify what—if anything—most Canadians can agree on, and create an all-inclusive definition of health that would be acceptable for each person regardless of his or her age or circumstances in life.

In her opening remarks to the finalists in the competition to design an American health system, Kathleen O'Connor said that "You can't design a ship until you know it has to float." This struck me at the time because it is the essence of what I have learned over my years of trying to reform health care policy. The best policies in the world will not be successful if there is not a shared vision of the final goal. You must define the *what* before you start proposing *how to*. This chapter walks you through the many considerations in developing an all-inclusive definition of health for the information age.

Three Universal Assumptions About Health

I have suggested that there is no shared vision for our current health system. There is not even agreement among the stakeholders on a definition of health. We are continually bombarded with diverse opinions and statistics on our health system and how to fix it, but is there consensus on anything? As my research on health evolved over the years, I began to recognize three areas of agreement about health in Canada—the only three items I have found that most Canadians agree on:

- Health, health care, health support and a health system must be people-centred.
- We must protect our publicly funded universal health safety net as the basic level of care that all Canadians can access.
- The purpose of the Canadian health care system is to support the health of Canadians.

These may sound obvious, but recognizing them was an important first step. Until I was able to establish some common ground it was impossible to develop a model that all Canadians could embrace.

Health, health care, health support and a health system must be people-centred

Following the metaphor of the four pillars introduced in Chapter 1, *health* is what the individual patient wants, *health care* denotes the providers, and *health support* refers to all the support groups in a health system. This statement simply asserts that these stakeholders exist primarily because there are people with health needs. If for any reason the stakeholders are not directly or indirectly fulfilling a health need for an individual or group, then they are no longer compatible with the first aim of the system.

Although this assumption also seems obvious, Canadians must begin to understand that the goal of the current system is not always the health of the individual. Protecting a particular provider's rights, championing not-for-profit or for-profit systems, or winning elections: each can be the (unstated) non-negotiable goal and the patient must compromise his or her health goals to fit.

The *health system* refers to the legislation, policies and Acts that provide the direction and parameters for all stakeholders to achieve the health goals of Canadians. Like the stakeholders, the system was created only because there are people with health needs and so it, too, must centre on people. The need for compatibility and a shared vision by all stakeholders is critical to the success of the system.

We must protect our publicly funded universal health safety net

The commitment of our nation to guarantee all Canadians access to a universal level of health support has become an important part of what it means to be Canadian. Protection of this right is a fundamental concern of all Canadians. Canadians should be concerned, because unless there are changes in the system we are at risk of losing or severely compromising this essential element of our social fabric.

The purpose of the Canadian health care system is to support the health of Canadians

There are two key words in this assumption: *support* and *health*. If the purpose of the system is to support the health of the people, then it is essential that all stakeholders in the health system share a clear understanding of what support means and what it is that we are supporting. Without this understanding there is no clear vision—all the stakeholders act on their own definitions of the purpose rather than fulfilling a shared vision. Again, if there is no alignment of purpose on the team's goals, then it is extremely difficult to achieve them. And so it is important to clarify the terms *support* and *health*.

What is Support?

With the exception of emergency or life-support care, no individual, government or group can buy, give or legislate health for an individual. As health issues and treatment options become more and more complex, it is impossible for a third party to impose a universal solution for any health issue. A third party can provide support only to help an individual overcome the barriers to achieving his or her health goals. For example, the governments' role should be to establish the legislation, acts and policies that support the health of the people without imposing limitations.

Health providers have a saying that sums this up neatly: "There is nothing a doctor can do that will overcome what the patient will not do." Although every provider probably starts off trying to change the

There is nothing a doctor can do that will overcome what the patient will not do.

world and save the people, the reality that all they can do is to offer support is something all providers are quickly forced to accept.

Informed Canadians believe in universal support, but not in the same way we did in the 1950s and 1960s when Tommy Douglas was envisioning a health system. The expectations and goals then were much simpler. Canadians wanted to ensure that all citizens had access to basic emergency and illness care, and that people did not go bankrupt trying to obtain these services. Our expectations were realistic and we appreciated the support this gave us.

Today the goals are very different, the type of support needed to achieve the goals is very different and our expectations are very different. For example, 40 years ago a goal of the evolving system was to treat disease or acute illness, whereas today the goal goes beyond illness and is more often the management of chronic illness or degenerative disease. Because of exponential growth in research and technology, the treatment options are almost unlimited.

There must be a way to support all Canadians with a defined level of care without compromising individual health goals and creativity. The sooner our governments accept this challenge and realize that a

The sooner our governments accept this challenge and realize that a public health safety net is only one of many support systems, the sooner Canadians will move from being victims of an over-burdened publicly funded support group to being the beneficiaries of a multi-faceted health support system.

public health safety net is only one of many support systems, the sooner Canadians will move from being victims of an over-burdened publicly funded support group to being the beneficiaries of a multi-faceted health support system. The sooner governments develop legislation that allows choice, the sooner we will begin to design a health ship that will float.

The current health system imposes universal measures to

treat illness rather than supporting the health of the individual, and as the difference becomes more apparent, the challenges to the existing system will increase. *Government's role is to offer universal support. The individual's role is to determine how best he or she can use the support to address personal health needs. It is this choice of how we use the support that is one of the missing pieces for the transition to people-first health care.*

What is Health?

My professional training since graduation in 1973 has been extensive, but I experienced some of my most meaningful learning experiences at the Pankey Institute for Advanced Dental Education in Miami, Florida. Dentists from around the world go to the institute for one-week sessions to develop their professional skills, not only as dentists, but as citizens who are expected to be effective parents, team leaders and community leaders and, through it all, stay in balance.

During one of my first weeks at the institute, Dr. Harold Wirth, a founding member, mentioned a quotation from the American motivational author Napoleon Hill that has stayed with me: "What the mind can conceive and believe it can achieve". Dr. Wirth stressed that if we as health care professionals want to help our clients become healthier we must inform, empower and support them in their journey to achieve their goals: provide information so they can conceive personally relevant health goals, empower them with options for care so they believe it is possible, and finally support each person as he or she searches for ways to achieve their goals. This seems an obvious way to help, but so much of health care is still focused on the quick fix.

> *...if we as health care professionals want to help our clients become healthier we must inform, empower and support them in their journey to achieve their goals*

First, if health providers take the time to get to know their clients and develop a trusting relationship respecting their individual values and goals, they will have built the foundation needed to influence their clients' health in a very different way.

Second, if providers openly share information, help people clearly understand their options and help them find realistic ways to implement their options, then a personally relevant definition of health for the patient becomes a reality.

And third, if the health teams support people as they deal with the bumps along the road of our personal health journeys, the trusting relationship grows.

When the mission for a health team includes those three steps, your health journey is off to a very positive start. Once you have a personally relevant definition of health and a plan to achieve your goals, the transition to optimal health moves from an impossible dream to an achievable goal.

The idea of providers taking an *informing*, *empowering* and *supporting* approach to patient health care made a lot of sense, and has led me on a journey to develop an informed and empowered people-centred model for care in my practise—one that leads to a new definition of health.

Perhaps the best internal test of the care provided by all health teams is whether they would do anything different if the person was a family member. My proposal for reforming the health system is based on the type of system that would best support those I love most.

A Pyramid of Health

In this age of information and empowerment, there has been a fundamental change in our expectations. We've gone from the treatment of disease and illness to what I would now call supporting a personally defined balance of health. While trying to understand and explain this transition from disease to health, I discovered a close relationship between Abraham Maslow's hierarchy of needs and my vision of health. Maslow, an influential psychologist, argued that all people have basic needs and that as our needs are met, new needs emerge such that we are always striving for more or better.[22]

He proposed that human beings are motivated by unsatisfied needs, and that certain lower needs must be satisfied before higher needs can be satisfied. He believed that people are generally trustworthy, self-protecting and self-governing, and that we tend toward growth and love. Violence is not an inborn trait of human nature. Rather, violence and other evils occur when human needs are thwarted. In other words, people who are deprived of basic needs such as safety may defend themselves by violent means.

According to Maslow, there are general types of needs (physiological, security, belonging, and esteem) that must be satisfied before a person can act unselfishly: "As long as we are motivated to satisfy these cravings, we are moving towards growth; towards self-actualization. Satisfying needs is healthy, while blocking gratification makes us sick or evil." The need for self-actualization is "the desire to become more and more of what one idiosyncratically is, to become everything that one is capable of becoming".[23] In a nutshell, we are all "needs junkies" with cravings that must and should be satisfied.

Graphically Maslow created a pyramid to represent his hierarchy of needs:

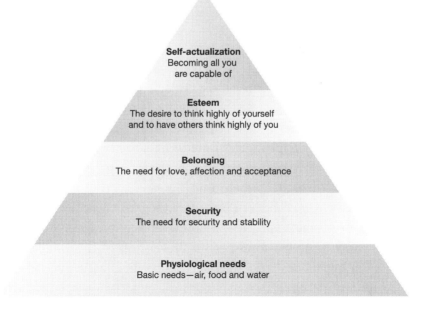

Fig. 2.1. Maslow's hierarchy of needs

As I thought about my life health experiences, five distinct levels of health and a transition stage emerged that correspond closely to Maslow's hierarchy of needs:

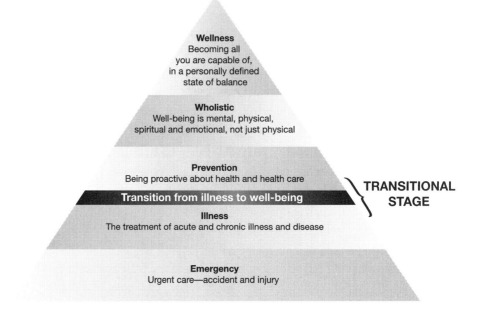

Fig. 2.2. The pyramid of health

Parallel to Maslow's model, we are also motivated by unsatisfied health needs, and certain basic health needs must be satisfied before we can move to higher needs. When we did not have basic emergency care, then we truly appreciated a medicare system that provided universal access to this care. Once the emergency needs were met, we began to focus on acute and chronic illness.

We have now reached a point where the two lower levels of health needs are being met, and we demand something more. We want to stay well and enjoy life-long health. Prevention of illness and emergencies is a logical next step to ensure a predictable quality of life.

Although life circumstances such as an accident or heart attack can quickly put a person back into the emergency or illness levels, each person's health journey generally progresses from one level of the pyramid to the next—from *emergency* and *illness* to *prevention*, then *wholistic* and finally to a level of health that we define as *wellness*, which corresponds to Maslow's self-actualization. The levels of the pyramid can be grouped into the three stages of our journey to wellness. The first two levels make up the illness stage, followed by a transitional stage; the top three levels represent the stage of well-being. Together they form an all-inclusive health pyramid. Understanding these stages will help us understand the differences between our current illness system and a vision for a health system.

The Illness Stage: The First Two Levels of The Health Pyramid

The emergency level

Emergency care, like Maslow's physiological needs, addresses the very basic health needs of the individual: urgent care and crisis management, including pain, swelling, bleeding, life-threatening illness, accident, trauma and mental and emotional urgencies. Canadians have agreed to pool our resources and attempt to help all individuals deal with these unfortunate but inevitable crises in life.

The problem is agreeing on what constitutes an emergency, what should be covered universally and how to define what is covered. The emergency level of health requires the most external intervention and is often the most expensive. It involves the most professional expertise, time and energy. This is the level of care that all Canadians want to support and this is the level of care that our system supports the best. There is unanimous agreement that it must be included in the universal health safety net; there has never been a consensus, however, on how much people can expect the system to provide universally.

The illness level

This level of health includes acute and chronic disease or illness. Although not usually life-threatening in the short term, this level of health problem seriously compromises the ability of a person to function effectively in society. Disease and illness demand a high level of professional expertise and are very costly to treat.

Most people agree that many health issues that are considered illness or disease should be included as part of the health safety net. As disease moves farther from emergency, it becomes more subjective, personalized and increasingly difficult to manage universally. As we examine the complexities of illness care in this technologically advanced age, it is apparent that there is no universally accepted formula for treating illness, and there are no limits to a great deal of illness care. But what levels of care are actually covered by the so-called universal, publicly funded system? Where do each Canadian's rights end and responsibilities begin?

Regardless of how much we invest in illness, everyone eventually gets sick and dies. Accepting this reality means that we must establish limits, and it challenges one of the basic premises of the current system: that we can successfully provide universal support for illness.

Regardless of how much we invest in illness, everyone eventually gets sick and dies. Accepting this reality means that we must establish limits, and it challenges one of the basic premises of the current system: that we can successfully provide universal support for illness.

Throughout this book I will be suggesting that we have to change the way we look at things. For example, a more realistic objective would be to provide a defined level of support for illness care that is universally accessible, and accept that people must assume responsibility for any care beyond this defined level. This is nothing new, but accepting it will be a huge shift in the way people think. Whether it is a waiting list, an 85% hip, or a private hospital bed, there are limits to what the system has provided. Informed people are accepting their responsibilities and making choices, even if it means going to Quebec or the United States where the desired service is offered. The next step is to design the system around this reality, rather than pretending it does not exist.

The Transitional Stage

To move beyond illness we must cross a threshold. Before the information age, very few people developed the tools to move beyond this threshold by design rather than accidentally. Two factors or catalysts are required to cross it: information and empowerment.

As we become informed about options and realize that it is often unnecessary to be ill, then we can begin to make choices to support our health.

As we become empowered with this information, we can choose to cross the threshold and begin to pursue and support health rather than treat or react to illness. One thing is certain: governments can't give or buy us a ticket to help us cross it.

The aim of the health system should be to support people so they can cross the threshold—to eliminate barriers to information and empowerment so that all individuals have the opportunity to move beyond illness to the various levels of health, if they so choose.

To make this transition requires that health stakeholders change the way they look at things. These changes are outlined in detail in the next chapter as the principles of health.

Personal Well-being: The Next Three Levels of The Health Pyramid

The prevention level

Preventive health is the first stage in the transition from treating sickness to supporting health. Corresponding to security needs in Maslow's hierarchy, the prevention level is a proactive level of health. Although there are exceptions such as vaccinations or water-purification programs, prevention usually involves much more than providing a treatment—it involves behavioural change. Whether it is brushing your teeth, exercise, diet or lifestyle changes, these are all examples of preventive measures that require a change in behaviour.

The challenge for a public insurance support program is how to support the intangible and indefinable skills required for behavioural change. There is no prescription that can be filled out to provide prevention. Care, skill, judgement, listening, communication, values clarification, empathy and understanding are all essential tools of preventive health counselling and care. It is at this level that measuring and

Successful prevention is ultimately determined by the patient.

managing become very difficult. Regardless of how effectively these intangibles are provided, successful prevention is ultimately determined by the patient. After we cross the threshold, dependency on material support begins to decrease dramatically. The inability of the current system to recognize and reward these intangibles is a major barrier to implementing prevention as an essential part of an effective and sustainable health system.

The wholistic level

Health in the emergency and illness levels is viewed primarily as being either a physical or mental issue. At the wholistic level, health is much more: Health becomes a personally defined balance of mental, physical, spiritual and emotional well-being. As we move through the different ages and stages of life, the balance will change. For many people—including me— physical health and aesthetics were extremely important in the younger years. As I have aged there have been many changes in my self-defined balance. Although physical health is always important, I find that emotional and spiritual health are becoming much more of a priority.

"Holistic" was the original spelling when Jan Smuts coined the term in the 1920s. I prefer the alternative spelling with a "w" because we are focussing on the well-being of the whole person.

The wellness level

Wellness is the level of health paralleling Maslow's concept of self-actualization. Self-actualized people are informed, empowered and independent. Each is responsible for the self, supports others and often can make the greatest contribution to the well-being of the whole community. Well people are aware of their personal journeys to being well, and are excellent coaches for others struggling to achieve their health goals. As the "beloved physician" St. Luke recorded, "Give, and it shall be given unto you".[24] Well people are most able to give back.

I believe that the following definition of wellness best expresses the ultimate goals of a people-centred system: *you are well if you embark on and accept responsibility for a personal journey to become all you are capable of, with a personally defined balance of mental, physical, spiritual and emotional health, and accepting the realities of life at the time.* This concept of wellness includes several important elements:

...you are well if you embark on and accept responsibility for a personal journey to become all you are capable of, with a personally defined balance of mental, physical, spiritual and emotional health, and accepting the realities of life at the time.

- *embarking on a journey:* We cannot be passive and be well. We have to be active. Nobody can give it to anyone else. Your own involvement is a critical step in what enables you to be well.
- *accepting responsibility:* It is impossible for anyone to be a self-proclaimed victim and be well. Until we accept personal responsibility and stop naming and blaming people and circumstances outside our control, wellness is not possible. You have to learn to accept and play with the cards you are dealt and find ways to improve your hand.
- *a personal journey:* Only the owner of the body can define the steps in the journey. No government, provider or other individual can assume this role. If they do, then wellness is not achievable. There is no end-point to wellness, because each of us is always capable of becoming more. It is a self-defined life-long journey.
- *becoming all you are capable of:* Wellness is that level of health when you consciously pursue optimal health based on your capabilities at the time. Wellness is self-defined.
- *personally defined balance of mental, physical, spiritual and emotional balance of health:* Each of us is unique and has a unique set of life circumstances. People either consciously or unconsciously define their personal balance of health. Wellness can only occur when this becomes a conscious act.

- *accepting the realities of life:* Wellness cannot occur until we accept our life circumstances (time, energy, and social and financial realities) and begin the process of moving on from that point. Some of the most graphic examples of our ability to cope with reality are the many stories of sports, military, spiritual and political leaders who came out of poverty and privation. Materially or physically they had very little to work with, but they accepted the reality of where they were and embarked on a journey to become all they were capable of being. Similarly, some of the least well people have unlimited material wealth and resources, but have failed to accept responsibility for a personally defined health journey. Acceptance of what, who and where we are in life is fundamental to wellness.
- *a given time:* Your definition of what you are capable of is unique, and it also varies at different times of your life. Living in the present is fundamental to wellness. Current reality, not the past or future, is where wellness begins.

This definition is particularly appropriate because it is achievable by everyone. Wellness is (and should be) a personal choice, not something that only the wealthy or privileged can achieve. Wellness is not dependent on physical attributes or genetic background. Wellness is a state of well-being that is determined by how we use what we have, rather than attempting to get something we don't have or what a third party believes we should have. You cannot buy wellness—you must earn it by using the tools you have.

> **Wellness is (and should be) a personal choice, not something that only the wealthy or privileged can achieve.**

I have often stated that one of my goals is to die well. Although a person may be physically ill, wellness is still an achievable goal even to the point of death. In a recent television contest to determine the greatest Canadian, the legendary Terry Fox was nominated. Early in life he was afflicted with cancer, and although he lost his leg he decided to make a difference by attempting to run across Canada with an artificial leg. Instead of complaining about what he didn't have, he decided to become all he was capable of with what he did have. Despite his death at a young age, he has left a legacy that continues to be the greatest fund-raiser for cancer research in the world. People like Terry Fox died well, by this definition. There was nothing our treasured illness system could do for him, but in spite of all his physical hardships he fulfilled his journey to wellness.

40 Years of Dramatic Change

The definition of health and our expectations for health care have changed dramatically. One of the major issues for any health support system is change. The type of support required to treat illness in the 1960s or even 1984 when the current *Canada Health Act* was written is very different from that required to support health in the 21st century.

Problems arise when a support group commits to universal care for one definition of health, but the definition and expectations all change. The problem becomes a crisis when there is no leadership to recognize the changes and revamp the system.

Problems arise when a support group commits to universal care for one definition of health, but the definition and expectations all change. The problem becomes a crisis when there is no leadership to recognize the changes and revamp the system.

Health in the 1960s

Health care providers in the 1960s were beginning to manage chronic disease and focus on health promotion, but the system was primarily focused on emergency or illness care for a patient who was poorly informed and very appreciative of any assistance he or she received. The care was concentrated on the treatment of physical illness and was easily measured and managed, and patients and providers had realistic expectations. There was much less chronic care and people were much less aware of the difference between treating symptoms or causes. The system was doctor-centred and most people accepted without questioning the options the doctor offered.

Health in 2005

Compare this with health and health care in 2005 when acute illness is not necessarily the primary concern. The care is increasingly focused on treating chronic disease or managing degenerative diseases that are life-long problems. A rapidly growing number of people are informed clients or consumers who are very aware of the many health options and want to play an active role in their continuing treatment. They appreciate support but are much more demanding. Physical health is only part of the expectations: they are also looking for spiritual, mental and emotional well-being. Care is often patient-driven, and the informed individual no longer accepts a paternalistic approach from an authoritarian doctor.

The following figure suggests in a simplified way the differences in some of the main tendencies and trends in medical care between the 1960s and today:

1960s	2005
Treat disease	Support all levels of the health pyramid
Treat patients	Work with patients, clients, consumers and users
Provide acute and emergency care	Expectation of life-long health
Primarily physical	Mental, physical, spiritual and emotional well-being
Treat infection, disease and illness	Manage degenerative disease and illness
Paternalistic	Patient-driven

Fig. 2.3. The focuses of health care in the 1960s and in 2005

We are attempting to support more complex and more costly long-term problems for much more demanding clients with a system that is struggling to maintain (rather than expand) support and is resistant to information, change and growth. If that is not a prescription for failure, then I don't know what is.

No wonder those who understand the complexities of health support say it is time to think outside the box and develop a system that can support the realities of a contemporary definition of health.

What exacerbates the problem is that there seems to be no

We are attempting to support more complex and more costly long-term problems for much more demanding clients with a system that is struggling to maintain (rather than expand) support and is resistant to information, change and growth. If that is not a prescription for failure, then I don't know what is.

leadership that will name the problem, openly consider the possible solutions and design a plan to achieve the goal.

Towards a People-Centred Definition of Health

It is clear to me that any definition of health must embrace three fundamental factors: *change, people* and *information*. Each highlights the fact that the current system is not founded on an all-inclusive definition of health.

Embracing change

The definition of health must be dynamic and changing. Never again can we go 20 years without an open review of the system. Virtually all aspects of health have changed: who can deliver care, who should deliver care, where it can be delivered, what services can be offered, and when, where and how they can be delivered. All of these changes would have an effect on any support system, but for one that claims to provide universal excellence, this is a serious management problem.

These changes are occurring at an ever-increasing rate because of research, technology and education, and there is no sign that change will slow down in the future. The next definition of health must embrace change.

Embracing information

The accelerating rate at which health-related information is being generated is affecting all aspects of our health system. New techniques and technologies result in increased options. As we become better informed we become aware of what is possible. When the system is unable to keep pace with the options we become dissatisfied. Information is one of the driving forces behind the need for change and is one reason alternative models are forming. We need a definition of health that is flexible enough to adapt to the new information that is available to each Canadian.

Embracing people

The definition of health for a patient-centred system must support every one of us, regardless of our life circumstances or background. It is no longer acceptable to define health or establish limits for health care based on public opinion polls or political philosophies.

In our cosmopolitan society, health can be defined differently not only for different regions of the country but also for different socio-economic groups, ages and cultures. The definition of health even changes for each individual as his or her circumstances in life change. Each of us has the right to define health based on our own personal values, and health support groups—be they public, private, for-profit or not-for-profit—must support us without infringing on our basic rights.

If our system is embracing all people, then health care also varies. The system was designed around traditional western medicine, but many other forms of medicine are widespread in Canada, including acupuncture, osteopathy, chiropractic and homeopathy to mention a few. A people-centred system must recognize freedom of choice and diversity in peoples' backgrounds and experiences. Any group has the right to distinguish the focus of its particular form of support, and this issue can no longer be ignored by governments who are managing a publicly funded support group that claims to be universal.

Some of the healthiest, most inspiring people are the terminally ill—not because they are physically well, but because they are mentally, spiritually and emotionally at peace with who and what they are. Being healthy is about becoming more knowledgeable about our bodies and minds and accepting responsibility for our own well-being. It is becoming independent as a unique and special person instead of being dependent on a system. A healthy person is empowered and creative in using all the available support systems to find ways to achieve his or her own health goals. Our new definition of health must embrace the unique qualities of an empowered and informed people.

The Transitions From Illness to Health

The expectations of a health system change as people cross the threshold in our pyramid of health from illness to well-being. As we become more informed and empowered, many transitions occur. Informed and empowered people do not approach life in the same way. Figure 2.4 (next page) shows several of the transitions as we move beyond the threshold.

What is the Current Definition of Health?

This is one question that people must begin to ask their health leaders. It is curious that very few stakeholders have a definition of health that is current. In my presentations to various provider, political, patient and business groups, I often ask for their definition of health. Although many individuals can put together a personal definition, the major health organizations and government agencies have not reviewed their definitions of health in many years.

The most common response is some variation of the World Health Organization (WHO) definition that was set out in the organization's first constitution in 1948 and remains essentially unchanged: "Health is a state of complete physical, mental and social well-being and not merely the absence of disease and infirmity." But this definition is very awkward because no one has ever achieved complete mental, physical and social well- being.

It is interesting that the principles of the WHO constitution also affirm that, "The enjoyment of the highest attainable standard of health is one of the fundamental rights of every human being.... The achieve-

Tolerating illness	Experiencing well-being
Reactive: responding to external circumstances that are beyond our control	Proactive: plan before illness strikes
Dependent: requiring external intervention and support.	Independent: internally driven and managed. External support helps but success is client driven.
Physical: very focused on physical or mental illness	Wholistic: focused on mental, physical, spiritual and emotional health
Tangible treatment: dependent on things—drugs, surgery, life support, x-rays, equipment, hospitals, etc. Success can be measured by a third party, and the outcomes are based most often on what the third party does rather than by what the patient does	Intangible treatment: support moves beyond a tangible focus and is more dependent on communication, listening, empathy, care, trust, relationships, clarification and values coaching. Success can only be measured by the individual. Outcomes are most often dependent on the individual rather than the type of equipment or the sophistication of the facility.
Crisis management and clearly defined standards with few options.	Long-term management with many options
Acute care	Life-long care
Treating illness	Managing health issues
Large financial investment and the quick fix	Smaller financial investment short-term but larger long-term (time and energy) investment on the part of the patient—a life-long commitment
Paternalistic: doctors are all-powerful and third-party support groups are in control. They both rescue petients and buy health.	Patient-driven: the patient is all-powerful. Third parties support the patient, and health is dependent on how effectively the individual and the support team work together.
Fearing physical illness	Embracing the fact that physical well-being is only one aspect of health and not necessarily the most important. It is possible to die well.

Fig. 2.4. Differences between tolerating illness and experiencing well-being

ment of any State in the promotion and protection of health is of value to all."[25] From this clause we could assume that any government would be in violation of this basic right if it failed to promote or protect the right of all people to be all they are capable of, given what is attainable. The question remains as to whether any government has the right to dictate what is attainable based on the economic realities of the government.

Another interesting fact is that Canada hosted a WHO meeting in 1986 and developed the *Ottawa Charter for Health Promotion*:

> Health promotion is the process of enabling people to increase control over, and to improve, their health. To reach a state of complete physical, mental and social wellbeing, an individual or group must be able to identify and to realize aspirations, to satisfy needs, and to change or cope with the environment. Health is, therefore, seen as a resource to everyday life, not the objective of living. Health is a positive concept emphasizing social and personal resources, as well as physical capacities. Therefore, health promotion is not just the responsibility of the health sector, but goes beyond healthy lifestyles to wellbeing.[26]

I encourage you to consider how the current system is implemented and whether it supports this Canadian-developed charter. Aspects of it seem congruent, but the concept of reaching complete physical, social and mental well-being means that health is unachievable. Consequently we would have to question whether it is an appropriate goal for a health system if there is a guaranteed 100% failure rate.

An All-inclusive Definition of Health

The challenge is to find a people-centred definition of health that embraces both sides of figure 2.4—tolerating illness *and* experiencing well-being—and all levels of the pyramid of health: one that embraces change, information and people, and that encourages information and empowerment so people can move beyond the threshold.

...health is a personally defined balance of mental, physical, spiritual and emotional well-being.

I propose the following people-centred definition of health: *health is a personally defined balance of mental, physical, spiritual and emotional well-being.*

With this definition, we have the basis for an all-inclusive health system. Regardless of where a person is on the pyramid of health, he or she has the potential of achieving health because it is personally defined. Wellness then becomes the ultimate goal of any health system.

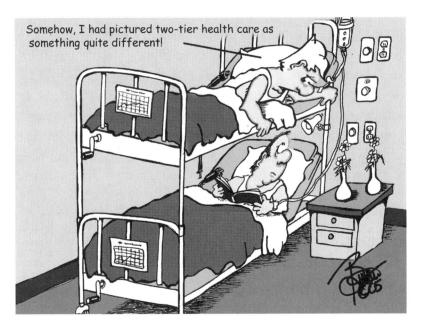

32 Million Health Systems

In only 20 years we have moved from a time when a universal health system seemed to be the ultimate solution to the crisis in health care, to a time when we are each capable of being the visionaries and architects of our own health systems. The role of the system is to support each person on his or her personal journey.

If health is a personally defined balance, we must have a system that can include 32 million definitions of health and potentially 32 million health systems, each personally defined and managed. This may seem overwhelming, but if our goal is to support health in a personal way, then the system that supports our goal will be very different from the crumbling system I outlined in Chapter 1.

The most significant fact is that despite all these changes in the way we look at things, the health safety net is still the fundamental building block that must be in place for all Canadians to begin our journey to wellness. We should be proud of where we are on our journey, but recognize that we have only just begun.

The next step is to investigate the principles on which a people-centred health system should be based.

SUMMARY—CHAPTER 2

In developing an all-inclusive definition of health, Canadians must take into account several considerations:

- the purpose of the system is to support the health of the people, and it is essential that support and health be defined
- there are five levels in an all-inclusive health pyramid: emergency, illness, prevention, wholistic and wellness
- there is a transition that occurs as people move from illness to well-being
- most aspects of health and health care have changed over the 40 years our health support system has existed, and they will continue to change
- health is a personally defined balance of mental, physical, spiritual and emotional well-being
- wellness is becoming all you are capable of with respect to your health
- there are potentially 32 million definitions of health (one for each Canadian) and these can change at any time; the challenge is to develop a system that supports each person as the visionary and designer of his or her own health program, rather than forcing the person to adapt to a system

CHAPTER 3

The Principles of People-Centred Health

People-centred health is based on six principles: individuality, personal responsibility, full information, choice, personally defined quality and accepting reality.

IN THE CURRENT CLIMATE of waiting lists, lack of choice and government-imposed quality, too many of us feel like victims of inadequate support, rather than the beneficiaries of a health-conscious society that is doing all it can to support its citizens. Most people in the world would appreciate any help they could get regardless of how long it took, but Canadians are frustrated—not because what they have is wrong, but because there is no alternative to waiting and no choice for services or quality except what the system is able to support. It is the controlling, manipulative way the system is implemented that makes Canadians feel like victims.

As I mentioned in chapter 1, the existing *Canada Health Act* is based on five principles (universality, comprehensiveness, portability, accessibility and public administration), but these are financial or insurance principles for a health financing system, not principles of health. When you implement a system on insurance principles then you ultimately fulfill insurance goals. But the purpose of the system is to support the health goals of the people. The next-generation health system must help us treat illness, yet it must also support health without denying us the right to accept and manage the best way we can. To achieve this we must implement principles that define and support an all-inclusive definition of health.

The Six Principles of Health

So far I have proposed the foundation for an information-age health system that will be patient-centred, support the health of Canadians, and embrace an all-inclusive definition of health. The next step is to identify the fundamental principles that enable people to move across the threshold from illness to well-being and become the managers of their own health. These six principles will be the benchmark for evaluating all aspects of the health system:

- individuality
- personal responsibility
- full knowledge and information
- creative choice
- self-definition of quality, and
- acceptance of reality.

1. Individuality

People who choose to move from being merely less diseased to being more healthy begin to recognize they are unique, and they celebrate their individuality. They accept that everyone is different genetically, behaviourally and in how they process information. People have different values and needs, and these change a great deal in each person at different ages, stages and circumstances in life. As a result, no one can define or predict a person's health needs—only the individual can determine the proper balance to meet his or her needs.

As we move through the five levels of the health pyramid from emergency to wellness, individuality increases. In emergency care there are many universally accepted solutions. We cannot argue that life support involves maintaining the basic physical needs of airway, breathing and circulation, and there are accepted research-based procedures to treat many injuries or illnesses. As you move to the prevention level, however, successful treatment depends more on behavioural change, and successful behavioural change is based on factors such as patient values and life experiences. At this level there are more options for providing support that will induce changes in behaviour.

With further movement to the wholistic and wellness levels, each person has the potential to be unique in a personally defined balance of mental, physical, spiritual and emotional well-being.

The principle of individuality creates an interesting problem: a patient-centred system must be inclusive enough to support 32 million personalized health systems that are unique to each Canadian and ultimately managed by him or her. As we begin to express our individuality there are fewer acceptable universal options. Figure 3.1 indicates the relationship of the five levels of health to increasing individuality.

The principle of individuality creates an interesting problem: a patient-centred system must be inclusive enough to support 32 million personalized health systems that are unique to each Canadian and ultimately managed by him or her. Health is a personally defined balance of mental, physical, spiritual and emotional well-being.

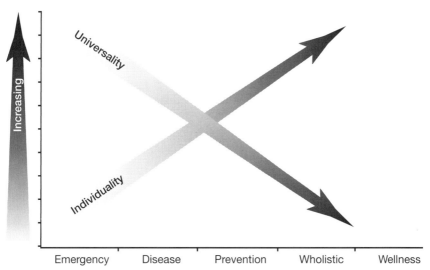

Fig. 3.1. Relationship of increasing individuality to the five levels of health

In the existing health system, the universality principle works according to the belief that if everyone can't have a particular treatment, then no one should. This affects how support groups work with patients. The role of the support group in a people-centred system will be very different. For politicians attempting to hang on to a health system based on the principle of universality, each person's uniqueness poses a major problem—another reason for changing the system.

2. Personal Responsibility

When we choose to move from being less diseased to being more healthy, we also come to appreciate that this is possible only if we accept responsibility for managing our own health. Every day in my dental practise I see real-life applications of the adage that "there is nothing a doctor can do that will overcome what the patient will not do." I have no doubt that no matter how good my diagnosis, treatment plan or treatment may be, if the patient does not do his or her part the treatment will fail. It is impossible for a person, group, government or provider to buy, give, legislate or prescribe health for someone else.

As we move through the levels of health, our responsibility and ownership increase while provider or support-group responsibility and ownership decrease:

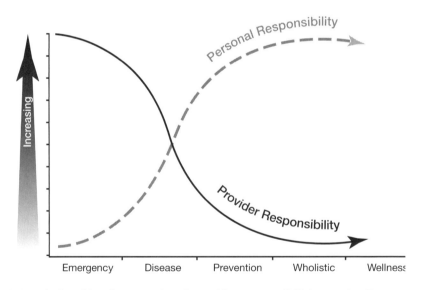

Fig. 3.2. Relationship of personal and provider responsibilities to the five levels of health

Responsibility and the 99+% Rule

When I make presentations about a people-centred approach to health reform, I am most frequently asked "what happens if a person does not want to or is unable to accept responsibility for his or her health?" I answer, "Who do you think is managing your health now, and who do you think is able to or would want to manage your health in the future?"

People believe that medical doctors or nurses manage the health of their patients, but in fact individuals manage their health for well over 99% of their lives without the assistance of

> *...individuals manage their health for well over 99% of their lives without the assistance of either doctors or nurses.*

either doctors or nurses. Consider the following facts as you face health challenges, and perhaps you will agree that it is time to change the way we look at things.

Health is a 24-hour-a-day job. What we eat, where we live, what we read, who we associate with, how much we exercise, our mental attitude, the environment, whether we smoke or drink, how much sleep we get, and most importantly what we do with the information or advice we are given—all these help to determine the quality of our health. Illness management by professionals is the exception for most people, and actually accounts for a small percentage of the average life span, but most people have never considered how small the percentage is. The best way to help people understand this issue is to review how much time is spent on illness care in the lifetime of the average Canadian, and how much of this illness care we already assume responsibility for.

There are several ways to estimate this, but one set of statistics we can work from is the number of providers and how much they work.

- There were 61,582 medical doctors in Canada in 2005.[27] Nearly 50% of these were specialists, but for this discussion we will assume that all are managing health care issues. If every one of these doctors worked 50 hours per week for 50 weeks of the year, this would mean that there was the potential of 2,500 hours per year for each doctor to manage health. Simple mathematics tells us that 61,582 doctors have about 154,000,000 hours to manage the health of the 32,000,000 Canadians entrusted to their care.

- This gives each person a maximum of 4 hours and 48 minutes with a physician in a year. Since there are 8,760 hours in a year, only 0.05% of the average person's life each year could be professionally managed by a doctor.
- In fact only about one-third of each doctor's time is spent in direct patient contact, so the actual average time for each Canadian to have doctor-managed care is probably less than 0.02% of the average Canadian's life annually.
- That leaves 99.98% for each of us to manage ourselves.

If you think that nurses change the statistics greatly, then consider these facts:

- Some 309,600 nurses and nurse practitioners worked in Canada in 2003 (the most recent year for which statistics are available).[28] If each nurse were to work 40 hours per week (even though many work part time) for 50 weeks of the year, then the average nurse would work 2,000 hours per year. This means there would be a potential of 619,200,000 working hours for nurses to manage the care of individual Canadians. That gives each of us 19 hours and 21 minutes annually during which a nurse could manage our health. If nurses only work one-on-one with their patients managing their health, this would account for 0.22% of the average person's life each year.
- According to nurses I have interviewed, only one-third of the average nurse's time (at the most) is spent with patients — less than 6 hours of health care management per year for each person.
- This means that 0.07% of the average person's life annually could be managed by a nurse.

Adding the 0.02% managed by doctors and the 0.07% managed by nurses, the total time that Canadians could have doctors and nurses managing their health is less than one-tenth of one percent. That is, *on average each of us manages our own health 99.9% of the time!*

But even this is optimistic if you consider the statistics on what we do with the information and services that professionals provide during their 0.1% of our lifetime.

It is well known among physicians and the pharmaceutical industry that there is less than 50% compliance with prescription drugs.[29] This means that patients don't fill the prescriptions, don't complete the prescriptions or take the medication incorrectly over 50% of the time. If we then consider the probable low compliance with nutrition and exercise programs, the theory that health providers manage a person's health becomes even more flimsy.[30]

Considering the 99+% rule and our poor compliance with our doctors' recommendations, it seems ludicrous for any politician or health professional to say that the average Canadian is incapable of managing his or her own health. The individual is the only person who can manage almost all health issues.

> *Considering the 99+% rule and our poor compliance with our doctors' recommendations, it seems ludicrous for any politician or health professional to say that the average Canadian is incapable of managing his or her own health. The individual is the only person who can manage almost all health issues.*

If these statistics are not enough to convince you that you are the manager of your own health, there is one final test. Simply ask your doctor whether he or she ever assumed responsibility for your health. You will find that there is indeed nothing a doctor can do that will overcome what the patient will not do.

3. Full Knowledge and Information

Healthy people never stop learning, growing and understanding themselves—they are life-long students of their personal health. People who move beyond disease care monitor their bodies and become familiar with their strengths and weaknesses.

...new currency of wealth is information and suddenly the industrialized world, which has a hierarchy based on material wealth, has been turned upside down.

In *The New Client*, Paul Hoffert discusses the power of information and its effect on society today: "The...new currency of wealth is information and suddenly the industrialized world, which has a hierarchy based on material wealth, has been turned upside down. The web is the bank of this new economy and everyone will have access to their own bank account.... As information becomes more available to clients, they become more powerful in transactions."[31] Health care will not escape the effect of this new currency. In the past, doctors too often did things to their patients without the patient's understanding why or how or even what the options were. In the information age, we are quickly becoming informed clients with whom teams of providers must work. Informed clients are unwilling to accept unconditionally what a provider does to them.

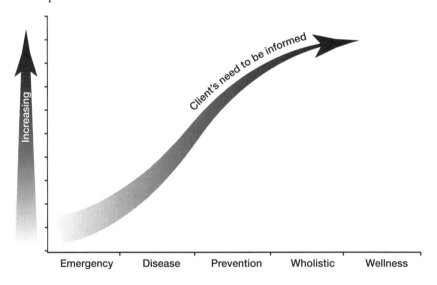

Fig. 3.3. Relationship of information needs to the five levels of health

Each level of the health pyramid requires an increasing level of knowledge and input from the patient. In emergency or life-support care, we are just bodies to work on. It is not necessary for us to know how to operate life-support equipment or how to set a broken leg, and it is not necessary to know why or how a particular drug works. A provider can often treat the symptoms of emergency and illness without our playing an active role. When we choose to treat the causes of illness or move beyond disease, our need for information, knowledge and understanding increases dramatically. The prevention, wholistic and wellness levels of health are possible only when we take control and make informed decisions. Figure 3.3 graphically suggests the increasing need for information as people move through the various levels of the health pyramid.

4. The Principle of Choice

Healthy people understand that there are choices to be made in any health issue, even if the only choice is to do nothing. As we move from emergency through the different levels of the health pyramid, the options increase. There are few choices in life support, but as we move to wholistic health and a personally defined balance, our options become limitless. To be healthy, each of us must participate actively.

Our desire for choice and options is increasing as our knowledge increases. At one time, we would have readily accepted the doctor's word and rarely asked for a second opinion. Today, we regularly research our symptoms or diagnoses on the Internet, and we arrive for appointments prepared to discuss the options. It is becoming a common occurance for patients to have discovered options of which their provider was unaware. As we embrace the principles of information and choice, the provider becomes a consultant, supporting an active participant rather than just a doctor treating a patient.

> *As we embrace the principles of information and choice, the provider becomes a consultant, supporting an active participant rather than just a doctor treating a patient.*

Clients who research health and seek options may frustrate providers who are not comfortable with being challenged on their diagnoses, but knowing our choices is an important step in our transition from being diseased victims to becoming self-actualized, well people. Figure 3.4 suggests the increasing number of choices as a person moves through the levels of health:

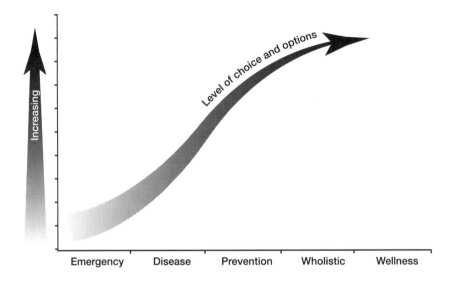

Fig. 3.4. Relationship of having choices to the five levels of health

5. Self-definition of Quality

The definition of quality changes more as we move up the levels of health. For example, there could be almost universal agreement on quality for emergency life support because it is a very physical and technical level of care. Quality can be determined by something as obvious as whether the patient lives or dies. Beyond life support, however, the quality of care is determined more by intangible services like the care, skill, judgement, empathy and communication skills of the provider. As we move from urgency to life-long care, we stop measuring quality by what providers do *to* us and start measuring it by what is done *for* or *with* us.

As we move from urgency to life-long care, we stop measuring quality by what providers do to us and start measuring it by what is done for or with us.

The quality of care provided by a nurse or nurse practitioner may be the main thing that many of us remember. Even though major surgery may have been performed by the surgeon, often the things that we remember most are the relationships and how support people reached out in a human and caring way to comfort us on our health journey. Figure 3.5 indicates our increasing ability to judge and define the quality of care as we move up the health pyramid:

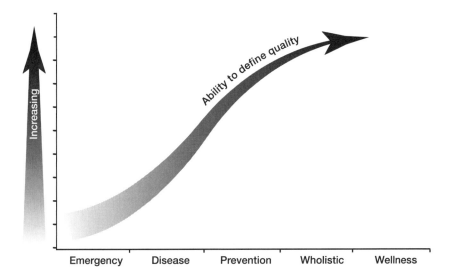

Fig. 3.5. Relationship of our ability to judge the quality of care to the five levels of health

6. Acceptance of Reality

Each of us has time, energy, social, financial and environmental realities that we must deal with as we pursue our personal well-being. We each have our own strengths and weaknesses in handling these pressures, but healthy people manage their strengths to overcome their weaknesses. Some of us have more time or energy, others have financial or social support, but regardless of the circumstances healthy people accept their reality and move forward. They do not see health as a competition—it is a personal challenge to become all we are capable of, based on our current realities. The healthiest people are not necessarily the wealthiest. The youngest and fittest are not necessarily the healthiest. Emergency and disease care are only the beginning of a life-long health journey.

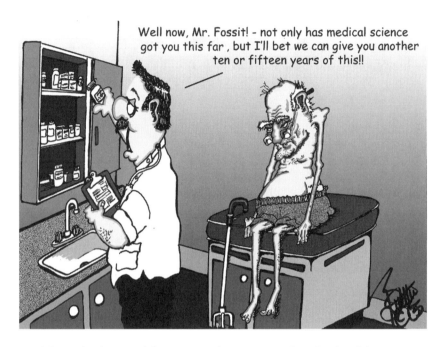

Although the wealthiest people may not be the healthiest, it is a truism that the wealthiest are often the least diseased.[32] The need for a universal health safety net will always be based on this. As we move to an all-inclusive health model, we must never forget that we do not want to revert back to the days when the poor and uninsured had dif-ficulties getting basic levels of emergency and disease care. These are the most expensive levels of health care, and the most demanding and time-consuming for the providers. The need for us all to pool our resources to provide the highest level of support possible for all Canadians is as real today as it was 40 years ago. The information-age challenge is to create a way to provide universal support by meeting this financial challenge without infringing on the other principles that allow us all to move beyond disease to health.

As each of us moves up the levels of health, the relative importance of some realities changes. For example, there is a decrease in the significance of financial support. Life support and major surgery are probably the most expensive of all kinds of care, but the financial costs of care decrease as people move beyond disease. At the level of prevention, behavioural change is essential. The material costs of successful preventive therapy are minimal, but the investment of time and energy by both patient and provider to achieve behavioural change is much greater than in disease or illness care. When a person moves to wholistic or wellness care the time, energy, social and environmental realities become increasingly significant, while the financial investment continues to decrease. With the financial support of a universal health safety net to assist us all with the expensive levels of care, we should all be able to manage the other realities to pursue our own personal balance. Figure 3.6 suggests the variations in the significance of these realities as we move toward wellness.

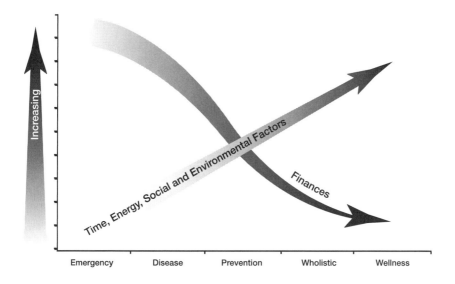

Fig. 3.6. Relationship of the realities of individual circumstances to the five levels of health

One Man's Search for Meaning

Perhaps one of the most moving stories about man's ability to be well, and to cling to the principles of health in almost impossible circumstances, is the story of a Viennese psychiatrist. Dr. Viktor Frankl was a Holocaust survivor, and his life story in his book *Man's Search for Meaning* is an incredible tribute to our desire to live and be well.[33] It is also a testimonial to the possibility to be well regardless of our life circumstances. Frankl managed to overcome the suffering and horrors of his imprisonment during the Second World War to become all he was capable of, even in the concentration camps.

Dr. Frankl determined that whatever else they took from him, they could never take his choice of attitude. Despite the humiliation and torture he stuck to his choice and would not allow circumstances to control his life, however difficult. He explained that in the lowest points of his incarceration, the only thing his captors could not take away was the sunrise and sunset. He blocked all else from his mind and focused on the fact that sunrise meant he had made it through to another day and sunset meant he had survived whatever he was meant to endure. He continued to be a survivor rather than a victim. He had maintained a personally defined balance based on his current reality—despite everything, he was well.

Applying the Principles of Health

Optimal health is not just the absence of physical or mental disease; it is a state of mind and body that only the person can define. It is the right of individuals to personally define their health, regardless of whether they are in their prime or on their deathbed.

Canadians have created an illness system around insurance principles and an insurance Act that is implemented so that it too often deprives us of our rights to apply the six principles of health. We have created a state of dependence that disempowers us.

This system is no longer acceptable. It is no longer acceptable that quality of care is determined by the financial limitations of Canadian governments that are over $794 billion in debt.[34] This type of system does not support health. It dictates health through legislation that controls the providers and limits everyone's options.

If we use the issue of the 85% hip from Chapter 1 as a test of principles, you can quickly see the problems with the current system.

Under the insurance principles of the existing *Canada Health Act*, the 85% hip is:

- universal (everyone can get one if they live longer than the waiting list)
- comprehensive (it is a necessary service and is included)
- accessible (all people have access to services, but there is no limitation on how long you will wait)
- portable (you can get it anywhere in Canada), and
- publicly funded (totally paid for by the insurance plan).

On the other hand, evaluating it from a health perspective and by the principles of health, the 85% hip does not:

- respect individuality (everyone is not treated as an individual)
- encourage responsibility (the patient is not even part of the process)
- inform the people (surgeons have given up telling people the facts because there is nothing they can do)
- support choice (options are not given because there are none, unless the government decides to free up more money)
- allow people to define quality personally (the government imposes quality based on age, public-opinion polls, lobbying and so forth), and
- accept the individual's circumstances or realities (the only reality is what the government is willing or able to do).

In Chapter 5 I will show how we can apply these principles in a report card for virtually all aspects of a people-centred system. In the meantime most aspects of the current system clearly do not support health principles, or inform, empower and support the individual as the manager of his or her own health.

It is up to each of us at the grassroots level to question the system, challenge the status quo, personally define what will best address our needs, and demand that the visionaries create a system that truly supports the health of all Canadians and the principles of health.

Unless most Canadians say we want something better, the system will never change. It is up to each of us at the grassroots level to question the system, challenge the status quo, personally define what will best address our needs, and demand that the visionaries create a system that truly supports the health of all Canadians and the principles of health.

SUMMARY—CHAPTER 3

What are The Principles of Health?

- the six principles of health, not insurance principles, must be the tools for evaluating all aspects of a health system
- regardless of our circumstances in life, the principles of health are controlled by each person
- health and wellness are possible for all people, not just the privileged
- on average each of us manages our own health 99.9% of the time

CHAPTER 4

A People-Centred Model for Health Care

A new vision for health care puts the individual at the centre, supported by the care provider or coach, many kinds of support groups, and innovative policies and legislation.

AFTER DEFINING HEALTH and the principles that support health, we can take the next step on our journey—to outline a practical working model for a people-centred vision of health care. This is a great challenge. No country has ever implemented a people-centred model, but Canada is perfectly positioned to be a world leader because we have a universal health safety net that guarantees access to basic illness care and we have the ability to inform and empower our people to move beyond basic health care. The question is whether we are committed to taking what we have accomplished and creating a system that is able to empower the individual as manager of his or her own health.

From what we have learned in the first three chapters, this new model should:

- be patient-centred
- support the health of Canadians as its primary purpose
- embrace change, information and people's diverse needs
- embody an all-inclusive definition of health
- incorporate the six principles of health, and
- reflect the Canadian desire for a universal health safety net.

A Graphic Approach to the People-Centred Model

My view of a model for care has evolved through research and consultation with colleagues, patients, friends and concerned persons over the years. It is most easily understood by visualizing the four pillars of health reform as four concentric circles, each representing one of the stakeholders: the individual, providers, support groups and the system.

1. The Inner Circle: The Informed Individual

A people-centred model must begin with the individual at the centre.

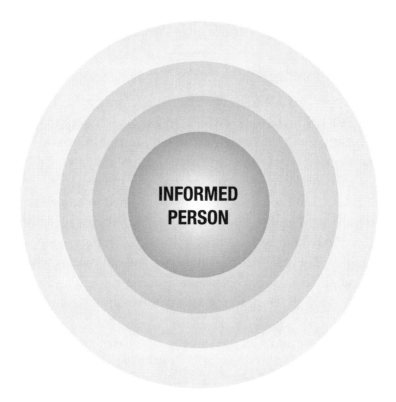

Fig. 4.1. The individual is at the centre of the people-centred model

Despite everything that society can provide or do to support health for us all, each of us is ultimately the centre of our own health system. To become healthier, it is important that each person accepts responsibility for the management of his or her personal health support system. Like the nucleus of a cell, the informed person is the control centre. The other levels exist to support the well-being of the nucleus, and are accountable to the centre.

> *Like the nucleus of a cell, the informed person is the control centre. The other levels exist to support the well-being of the nucleus, and are accountable to the centre.*

A people-centred model must be implemented in such a way that the patient always has the option to manage health and health care. This includes selecting the most appropriate provider or coach, the type of service, and how, when, where and why to use and pay for a particular form of support. Getting all parts of the health care system to understand and acknowledge this point may well be the greatest hurdle to overcome.

2. The Second Circle: The Provider or Coach

The next circle in the people-centred model is the primary provider or coach. This may appear to be similar to other health models, except that the coach may be (but not necessarily is) the doctor. Rather the coach is the support person who has established a trusting relationship with the patient and is most effective and efficient in helping him or her deal with a particular health issue. The concept of the coach is critical in moving to a people-centred model.

Traditionally the doctor has been the gatekeeper for primary care, and to this day the almost sacred doctor–patient relationship is too often the underlying reason for not looking at other health-coach options. A doctor–coach made sense 40 years ago when people viewed the system primarily as treating illness, because a medical doctor was the only person licensed to treat most illness. With a wholistic perspective of health, however, and with alternative health providers available for many health issues, the options for choosing a coach are expanding.

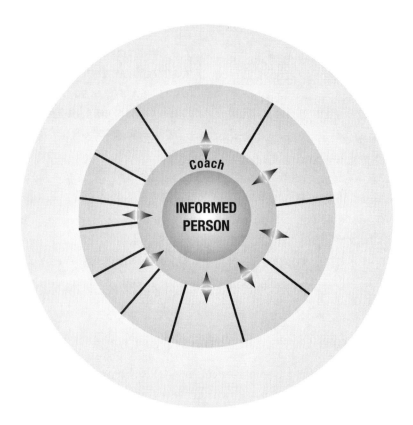

Fig. 4.2. The second circle: the individual has a trusting relationship with a
        provider or coach

Evolving from a doctor-as-God mentality
to an effective health team

After about six years in practise, my career in dentistry was not what I
had envisioned. I got tired of fixing teeth, and began to seek out ways
that I could care for people in what is now called a relationship-based
practise. Our dental practise gradually incorporated features of a people-centred model, and perhaps the most awkward part for me was
giving up my doctor-as-God status.

It was difficult for me to accept there were others on my team who
were more effective as the coach or central figure in many of the health
relationships with our clients. During the transition, for example, I dis-

covered that two people on our team were very effective listeners and communicators, and that everyone on our team had coaching and communication talents that were underused, or worse yet, not used at all.

I am like many health care professionals who love to diagnose and fix things, but we also like power and respect. Traditionally, doctors trained in Western medicine achieved their power and respect through the non-negotiable doctor–patient relationship, but they must be open to change. Let's examine each of these.

Diagnosing and fixing

There is a time and place for diagnosing and fixing. It is important, for instance, to act quickly in diagnosing and fixing pain, swelling, bleeding and other emergencies. This state of emergency is referred to as Code Blue in medical circles. If the ultimate goal is to treat emergencies, the doctor–patient relationship is often appropriate. If the ultimate goal is to treat emergencies so we can support health, the rules have to change. As we move away from treating symptoms toward finding and eliminating causes of disease, the roles of all members of the team (including the doctor) must change. Code Blue situations happen very rarely in medical practises, and virtually never in dental, chiropractic or other health environments. Why then do we have a whole model and system that function with a Code Blue emergency mentality?

It took me a long time to learn that if we want to move from simply treating illness to fostering health, it is important to refrain from diagnosing and treatment planning until the patient appreciates what the problem is, or that he or she even has a problem.

Achieving respect and power

There is a time, place and way to achieve respect and power, but using position or title to overpower and control are not the tools that work with an informed population. The way to gain power and respect is to empower and support others—the respect and power will come when it is deserved.

Empowering and supporting coaches or clients is not easy, and not something for which dental and medical schools prepare their students. In 1983 our dental team began team-development work-shops. The first team-development leader was a disaster and our whole team was ready to quit, so the first lesson is to find a facilitator who relates well to the team.

The second workshop was totally different. It was with Marion Balla, an Adlerian therapist and educator who was able to move the team (including me) quickly from total distrust of the team-workshop process to one of a trusting relationship. After 21 years we still meet with Marion at least once each year, and through her we have learned how to empower the team members (including the doctor) and to develop trusting relationships with one another. We then realized that we can use the same skills to empower our clients as the managers of their personal health.

We discovered that there must be consistency among how we treat ourselves, our team members and our clients. Developing listening and communication skills, problem-solving techniques and personal-development skills has changed both our working and personal lives.

Personally, I discovered that by empowering and informing those around me, I became more empowered and informed myself. As a paternalistic, know-it-all practitioner I had feared giving up control, but soon learned that my fears were unfounded. When each staff member is empowered to fulfill the role of coach, everyone gains respect. I have not lost respect as the leader of our practise, but gained respect in the eyes of the team and the patients, and I am much more effective as a diagnostician and treatment planner because I am able to focus much better.

When each staff member is empowered to fulfill the role of coach, everyone gains respect. I have not lost respect as the leader of our practise, but gained respect in the eyes of the team and the patients.

This philosophy of empowering others is not new in the business world, but it is new in the hierarchical world of health care. It is particularly novel in Canada, because the health system is not designed to enable and empower teams. The sooner we adopt an empowering and informing model for providing health care, the sooner all stakeholders will begin to experience the true rewards of a people-centred health system.

Other benefits

There are other positive effects of this team model. First, teams can help more people because there are more people contributing. Second, when team members take the extra time to help patients clarify realistic goals based on the patients' values, we find that people follow through on treatment plans because the plans are *theirs*, not the doctors'. (The relatively low compliance rates for drug prescriptions and exercise and diet programs may be related to the patients having played an insignificant role in the decision-making process.) When these two things occur there is a third benefit: the patient and the team are rewarded, not only materially but also personally and emotionally. The result is that patients learn to value medical staff because of their practical skills rather than their seniority or university degrees.

Coaches, also known as client co-ordinators or treatment co-ordinators, are listeners. They can quickly develop a relationship with a client that is different from the doctor–patient relationship. The experienced coach is like a confidant, and often there is a high level of trust in a relatively short time. The coach acts as an extra set of ears and eyes in the treatment, and is often the person the patient turns to when he or she has questions or needs clarification.

> *The experienced coach is like a confidant, and often there is a high level of trust in a relatively short time. The coach acts as an extra set of ears and eyes in the treatment.*

The importance of teams in creating effective and efficient systems

The role of the coach and the incentive to create teams are missing links in the current health system. By doctors' refusal to recognize the value and role that the people around them can fulfill, and their protection of the sanctity of the doctor–patient relationship, they are creating a doctor-centred system. Coaches are essential to making the system effective, efficient and accountable to the patient. By using less expensive team members effectively, we can also address some financial concerns. Moreover, if the system allows the provider to be rewarded for managing effective teams, we can have a situation where the patient, the team, the doctor and the insurer are all winners.

The transition to an empowered team is not easy

A patient-centred model is based on the six principles of health *(Chapter 3)*. Implementing a model that supports the health of the individual and respects and encourages each of the principles takes training, skill and time. Very few doctors take the time to reinforce these principles in their relationships and, quite frankly, few people can afford to pay the most expensive person in the office to help clarify which option is best or what quality of care addresses their needs.

Outside the public health system—where cost-effective and efficient alternatives are essential since the client is responsible for payment—many alternatives to the doctor as primary communicator have evolved. The use of empowered teams with client co-ordinators and treatment co-ordinators with excellent listening and communication skills are prevalent. It is time to explore more effective, efficient and less costly options and implement a system that encourages these options.

> *It is time to explore more effective, efficient and less costly options and implement a system that encourages these options.*

Health care is a business

Whether people like it or not, health care is a business. We all can see the results when the business of health is run as a free service with seemingly endless financial support. We see long waiting lists and shortages of doctors. We see a government constantly juggling and shifting financial priorities. Our free ride is coming to an end, and unless we create alternatives we will lose our beloved health safety net.

In business, if certain employees are specialized and it costs more for their expertise, it is good management to keep them in their specialties. Car dealers could never balance their books or be competitive if they managed the way the health care system does. They don't call in the mechanic to answer the phone and direct calls. Someone with communication and listening

...when the business of health is run as a free service with seemingly endless financial support. We see long waiting lists and shortages of doctors. We see a government constantly juggling and shifting financial priorities.

skills discusses options and begins the clarification process. It is a waste of time for mechanics to work outside their specialty.

If this simple business logic works for the very successful car industry, why don't we have a system that encourages us to apply these rules to the health industry? General practitioners specialize in diagnosing problems, planning treatment, and performing certain technical procedures. It is time to empower the team to make sure that the doctor invests most of his or her time in what only the doctor can do.

Is there a shortage of doctors or is it mismanagement?

Michael Rachlis and Carol Kushner note in *Second Opinion* that, "According to estimates, 80 per cent of all people that go to see physicians have nothing wrong with them that wouldn't clear up with a vacation, a salary raise or relief of everyday stress.

According to estimates, 80 per cent of all people that go to see physicians have nothing wrong with them that wouldn't clear up with a vacation, a salary raise or relief of everyday stress.

Only 10 per cent require drugs or surgery to get well, and the remainder have an illness for which there is no cure. This 80 per cent success rate helps to perpetuate the myth that physicians, both modern and ancient, have special healing power."[35]

In the same vein, a 1999 report by Ontario's Health Services Restructuring Commission found that 69% of the billings of general

...69% of the billings of general and family physicians for 1996–97 were for service fees that were within the licensed scope of practise of nurse practitioners, nurses and other (lower-cost) health care professionals.

and family physicians for 1996–97 were for service fees that were within the licensed scope of practise of nurse practitioners, nurses and other (lower-cost) health care professionals.[36] The exact numbers may be debated, but there is overwhelming agreement among the health care workers I have interviewed that someone other than the doctor could manage a high percentage of primary-care physician visits.

We need managers of health teams. If doctors are unable or unwilling to manage these teams, they should delegate the role to others. Too much of their time is currently invested in doing things that support staff could and should be doing.

A management model that encourages the whole health care support team to work together has clear benefits. By expanding the role of properly selected and trained members of the team, we would improve the system's ability to support greater numbers of people effectively in a caring and timely fashion. The quality time available to providers (including nurses and nurse practitioners) to invest with the patient would be increased, and overall there would be an enhanced level of care.

Quality of life is a major concern for providers

The expectation that the family doctor should work around the clock seven days a week and give up everything (including his or her own health) to fulfill the needs of patients is long gone. Quality of life is rightly a major issue for the medical doctor and all health-care workers. People who choose a career in health care are very caring and committed people, but they also have a life to live and each intends to live a personally defined balance of work, play, family and worship. Most are parents with families of their own, and their first obligation is to their family, not their practise.

The time is gone when the doctor was typically male, his wife was a mother with no career other than the family, and parenting was women's work. Enrolment in health care in most universities is now approximately 50% female, and it is not uncommon for there to be more women than men. Now round-the-clock doctors who are willing to give up everything else in life for their career are exceedingly rare. We must change the way we look at things and design a system that can thrive with these new realities.

The stress on a doctor who sees 50 to 70 people a day is overwhelming. That potentially 80% of them could be served by someone other than the doctor could go a long way in relieving doctors' stress, giving them time for a personal, family life as well as their career, and increasing their effectiveness in fulfilling the roles that only they can perform. This is not to say that the doctor would no longer be the visionary and leader for the care that is provided under his or her supervision. It is just that the doctor would be the last line of support whenever others are unable to manage the issue.

3. The Third Circle: The Support Groups

The third level of the people-centred model comprises the support groups. As you can see in Figure 4.3, there are many different kinds of support groups.

In the proposed system, the person and the coach would define health goals and then together go shopping among all the support groups to determine which options best address the identified needs. (The arrows between the various support groups and the coaching level indicate that members of particular support groups can assume roles as coaches, depending on the health issue and their relationship with the client.) There are always options for where or how to receive support. The universal health safety net continues to be a primary support system for the costly emergency and disease levels of care (and any other services it can afford to support), but it is only one of many support groups:

- *personal support:* The greatest support in any person's health is his or her personal support. By this I am referring to the 99%

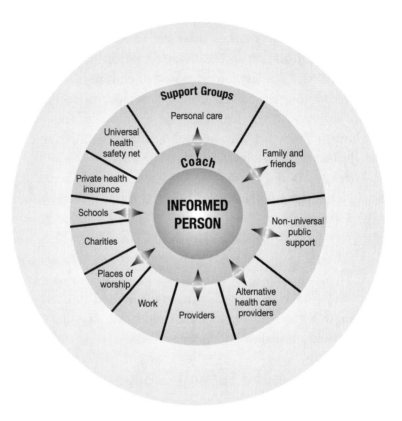

Fig. 4.3. The third circle: 11 kinds of support groups

or more of our lives when the average person is personally managing his or her own health and selecting the most effective ways to address our particular issues. The system must recognize and encourage this personal support to enable individuals to be the managers of their personal well-being.

- *family and friends:* The next largest support group is family and friends, and again the system must recognize and encourage this support. For much of our adolescent lives, most health concerns are managed by parents or guardians. Throughout life it is to family and friends that most people turn first for issues such as nutrition, fitness, and spiritual and emotional concerns.

- *non-universal public support groups:* We must not forget the many regional, community and provincial support groups that are publicly funded but are not universal. Groups for home care, child care, cancer support and so forth are all at least partially funded by public coffers, but often depend on user fees and private funding.
- *alternative health care providers:* This group accounts for a growing percentage of the health costs in Canada and must be recognized as an essential part of any future health systems. Chiropractic, optometry, physiotherapy, massage therapy, kinesiology, acupuncture and homeopathy, among many others are each recognized and valued by many individuals. Although the universal system is strained to the limits to provide emergency and illness care, developing a support system where people can use a portion of their support for services that best meet their needs rather than what is free of charge is something that we must consider.
- *support providers:* These are members of the support team other than the medical professionals who interact with the clients. Hospital auxiliaries, secretaries, assistants and volunteer groups offer a personal touch in an often hectic and over-committed system. These people often become coaches because they develop relationships and trust with patients and because they take the time to relate at a personal level.
- *work support programs:* Many employers have health-support programs and benefits that are increasingly important. For dental care, optometry, alternative medicine, and all the areas that the so-called universal system does not address, employee health benefits are a major factor in an individual's overall health management plan.
- *places of worship:* As we begin to take a wholistic approach to health, spiritual well-being can be a very important aspect of the journey to wellness. Spiritual leaders tend to be in touch with members of their congregations or followers at a very personal level, and are often the support system for people who fall through the cracks of the formal system.

- *charities:* Charitable organizations play a significant role in the system, although they do not have universal funding and they focus on particular health issues.
- *schools:* To develop a generation of informed and empowered people who will choose to fulfill a significant role in managing their personal health, formal learning about health must begin at an early age.
- *private health insurance:* As the universal system is forced to accept the limits of its support and cuts back on services, the role of private insurance will become more appealing. Many people already subscribe to private insurance, and their numbers are almost certain to increase.
- *universal health safety net:* The existing system is the only support that claims to be universal and publicly funded. All other support groups are either private or a public-private combination, and each is specific to a particular group, age, sex or health issue.

In a people-centred model, the boundaries and rules for the support groups are defined by the needs of the individual person, instead of by the needs of a political philosophy or by public opinion polls. All support options are welcome as long as they do not violate the definition of health (discussed in Chapter 2) and the six principles of health (Chapter 3).

As people are informed about all the support options that exist, the notion that there ever has been—or ever can be— a universal health support system fulfilling the health needs of the individual is an unrealistic political promise that has no relationship to reality.

One thing is certain. As people are informed about all the support options that exist, the notion that there ever has been—or ever can be—a universal health support system fulfilling the health needs of the individual is an unrealistic political promise that has no relationship to reality.

The need to be informed

For the support groups to work effectively with a person and his or her coach, each of us must accept our role as a manager and quality-control officer. To do this effectively, we need information that only the support group can provide:

- Each of us must have a clear definition of what service is being supported. This includes who is covered, what is covered, where it can be received and how it is funded.
- Each of us must have a clear understanding of what fees are reasonable and fair for the services we need. We must have access to fee guides with the associated norms of treatment, costs and times (both wait times and service durations) for delivering care. Health care is not universal. Every procedure is different, depending on the patient and the provider, and we need to be aware of how our support providers are rewarded.

For a people-centred system to work beyond the threshold of illness care, it must have the ability to recognize and reward the intangibles such as listening, communication, the difficulty of treatment, skill, empathy and caring, to name a few. Only the patient can assess these services. For payment guidelines to be effective, it will be necessary for all providers to provide defined services for specified fees.

For example, it is not enough for a support group to announce that it financially covers an examination. The support group has the responsibility to specify a time frame as well as what would be provided. Individuals and their coaches need this information about each and every procedure, to assess whether the support fulfills the person's needs and to assess the quality and integrity of the support group. With this information and a trusted coach to help process the information, we have the foundation for an effective and efficient health system that is focused first on the needs of the individual, but rewards the provider appropriately based on the outcome for the patient—no more rewards based on averages or which code is used.

4. The Outer Circle: Management and Legislation

The outer circle completing the people-centred model includes the legislation, rules and guidelines needed to enable the inner three circles to operate within a new health system, without imposing on the rights and responsibilities of other participants.

THE PEOPLE-CENTERED MODEL

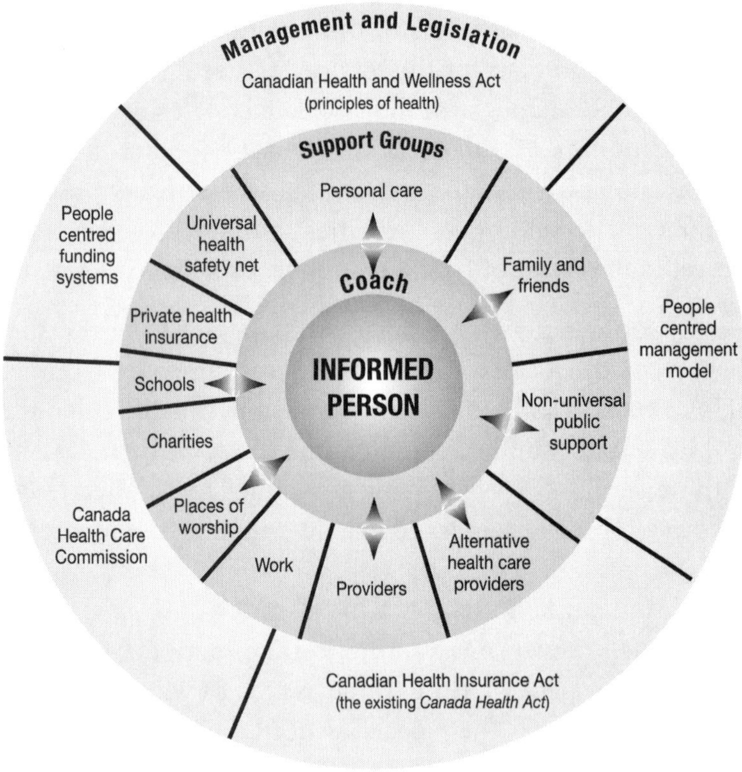

Fig. 4.4. The complete people-centred health system

To have a health system that puts people first, we must have legislation that supports this vision. The fact that we do not have legislation that defines and protects health rights and responsibilities for the individual is one of the biggest barriers to moving from disease care to wellness support.

The existing *Canada Health Act* should be renamed the *Canada Health Insurance Act* and harmonized with a new federal *Canada Health and Wellness Act*. Among other major provisions, the new Act would establish a people-centred management system, a people-centred funding system, and an independent Canadian Health Care Commission. Part II of this

> **The existing Canada Health Act *should be renamed the* Canada Health Insurance Act *and harmonized with a new federal* Canada Health and Wellness Act.**

book discusses each of these elements in detail, but it may be useful here to introduce the reasons for setting up a non-partisan commission:

- We need continuing health policy regardless of which party is elected. After each provincial and federal election there is often a new Minister of Health, which creates a state of uncertainty in all stakeholders.
- The system exists to serve the needs of Canadians, so it must be founded on a definition and principles of health that cross all political boundaries.
- Governments must support the health system and manage the financing for the universal health safety net. Like all support groups, they must implement the support in such a way that they respect the principles of health and are accountable to a new *Canada Health and Wellness Act* that legislates the guidelines for health in Canada.

With a non-partisan commission, we will have a system in which governments as support groups are finally accountable to something other than public-opinion polls. The commission in turn would be accountable to an Act designed to protect the health rights of individual Canadians, regardless of who was in power. Until this legislation is in place, the move from the paternalistic, government and provider controlled system to a people driven, informed and empowering health system can never occur. All of the great ideas we can come up with to make the system more responsive to our needs will go nowhere if the legislation and management do not support them.

The Health System Puzzle

The complete people-centred system in figure 4.4 includes the major pieces of the health system puzzle. The challenge is to get the pieces in the right place. Currently the *Canada Health Act* is the non-negotiable base around which all the other pieces (including the patient and provider) must function. It directly and indirectly dictates the quality and type of care provided. If the goal is to support the health of the people, then this must change. The Act belongs on the outer circle, and although it fulfills an essential role, it is limited in what it can do. It is time to stretch our minds and think creatively to get the pieces in the right place, so that each person is in the centre of his or her personal health system.

SUMMARY—CHAPTER 4

What is a people-centred working model?

- it is a very different working model that will support a people-centred definition and the six principles of health

- the patient is the nucleus of any people-centred model

- the concept of coach is fundamental to the transition to an informed and empowered patient model

- there are many health support groups and providers: the universal health safety net is only one support mechanism and can never be all things to all people

- we must change the way we look at legislation, and creative minds are needed to create a Health and Wellness Act that will encourage the evolution of our system from illness to health and empowerment

CHAPTER 5

National Goals

Canadians have much to celebrate, but we have only completed the first step of our journey to wellness. Our next challenge is to become leaders in developing the world's first people-centred health model.

The concept of designing a system around the individual is an idea that is long overdue. The first four chapters of Part I, *What Needs to Be Done*, have outlined the state of Canada's existing health system, suggested a new definition of health and the six principles of people-centred health, and offered a people-centred model for health care.

In this chapter I will review the pros and cons of the current system, establish six goals for the evolving health system and challenge the idea that health care is really our number one priority. The chapter concludes by outlining the national goals to be kept in mind when you read Part II, *How We Can Do It*, and presents a handy report card for assessing any proposals for health reform.

Summarizing The Pros and Cons of Where We Are Now

On the positive side, one of the most important accomplishments of our country in the past 40 years is that Canadians made a commitment as a nation to support the health of the people. This sets us apart from many nations and is still the number one concern of most people.

However, things have changed in 40 years and we must not only be willing to change the way we look at things but also to do something about it. There are aspects of illness and emergency care that can be a public issue and can be addressed by a national program, but what we once viewed as health and health care has changed. The definition of health, who can provide health care, who should provide health care, what services can be offered, the abilities of people to participate in their own care, the expectations of people and the options for care have all changed—but the vision for the system is mired in political and professional debate.

As we begin to view health from the perspective of the individual we are forced to accept that the current level and form of support is only the beginning. We begin to realize there are limitations to what the public can do to support the health of the individual, and that health is ultimately a personal responsibility, not a public responsibility. This is not to say there is not a public role, but there is only so much the public is able and willing to do.

Canadians have completed the first step on our nation's journey to the ultimate goal of wellness, but it is time to develop a system that moves beyond the treatment of illness to helping the people become all they are capable of, with a personally defined balance of mental physical and emotional well-being.

There are many problems. Under our current health care system we have:

- a health Act that is not a health Act—it is an insurance Act
- principles for a health Act that are insurance principles, not health principles
- an illness system, not a health system
- no universal definition of health and therefore no agreement on what we are trying to accomplish
- a system that is not universal now, never has been and never will be
- an unrealistic and unsustainable financial plan with no boundaries and totally unrealistic expectations of what is possible (we could invest 100% of our tax dollars and everyone would still get sick and die)

- a politically-centred and a doctor-centred system—one that is failing to meet the expectations of both politicians and doctors—but not a people-centred system
- a so-called universal system that is primarily focused on an increasingly limited range of Western medicine despite an endless variety of alternative providers and approaches to care
- a system that is too often managed and directed by bureaucrats from political, business and professional special-interest groups who are not accountable
- a government or provider-centred management model for the system rather than a people-centred management model
- a system that resists change
- a system that fails to accommodate the diversity of an increasingly informed and empowered population, and
- a "politically correct" system that has lost touch with the health needs of the people.

Our next challenge is to become leaders in developing the world's first people-centred health model.

What a difference an "e" makes: the difference between "car" and "care"

Although Canadians have repeatedly said that health care is our nation's number-one priority, do our actions support this view that we claim is a fundamental part of our identity?

During a skiing trip with a car-dealer friend many years ago, we got to talking about the differences in our careers and the distorted values our clients had as a result of marketing and the media. Afterwards I began thinking about what would happen if we had a *Canada Auto Act* that was designed the same way as our *Canada Health Act*. What political party would have a chance of getting elected if it decided to impose a comparable *Canada Auto Act*?

The Canada Auto Act

1. There will be a universal car.
2. No options will be discussed. No one is entitled to a fancier car

than the poorest person can afford or the government is will-ing or able to provide.

3. All carmakers are equal in quality: therefore the same price will be charged for the car, and the government will set the price.

4. The price is the same for each car regardless of the car's comfort, convenience, safety, fuel efficiency or aesthetics; and regardless of the location of the dealership and the time the dealer spends with the client.

5. If you get an option or a different level of service and the dealer accepts a payment for this option or service, he or she will be fined up to $10,000.

6. Although there is only supposed to be one level of car, wealthy athletes, car dealers, politicians and influential people inside the system can get a better quality of car. The only difference is that they don't pay extra for it (even though they can afford to pay more, it is illegal). The result is this select group get the better quality car, but we all get to pay for this service from our taxes.

7. If you are under a certain age, you may be able to buy a longer lasting car, but only if the politicians say so. People over a cer-tain age cannot buy a longer-lasting, better-quality car because statistically they are not going to live as long or require the improved quality.

8. If a different political party is elected, one of three things may happen: your choice of car may remain the same, it may be reduced in quality, or you may get a better quality car if the party decides to take money out of education or social program.

9. If there is an economic downturn or if interest rates go up on the public debt, the quality of car will go down (unless the government decides to borrow money from your children to pay for your vehicle, with no obligation to repay the loan).

Canadians cheerfully accept that every citizen has the right to invest in different colours, shapes, comfort or speed for a car as suits their unique needs, but just put an "e" on the end of the word and suddenly there are no options. Is *care* not as important or as complex as a *car*?

As a Canadian I believe that all of my fellow citizens should have access to a defined level of health care that is the best our governments are willing and able to offer. But if options exist that meet my needs better, and if the public system is unable or unwilling to provide the options, then it is time to create a system that gives people and their providers access to those options.

Our Health Goals As A Nation

I strongly believe that we can set six realistic health goals for the nation based on the assumption that Canadians want their system to support all levels of health including wellness, and not just treat illness:

1. to define health and the principles of health and to make these the basic conditions for future health policy
2. to inform, empower and support each individual as the potential manager of his or her own health
3. to provide a universal level of support and implement it in such a way that it does not violate the first two goals
4. to create an effective, efficient, accountable and sustainable health system that supports the health of the people
5. to accept that change is inevitable, that information can change, that people are individuals, and never again to go 20 years without re-evaluating our health system, and
6. to define the limits of what we as a nation are able and willing to do to support the health of the people, and to develop health policies that work within those limits.

We cannot continue to compromise all other social programs to fulfill the unrealistic goal of complete mental and physical well-being. A universal health safety net is something we are all proud of, but it is only the first step on a nation's journey to wellness. If we truly want to support all people in their personal health journeys, then the next generation's health system must be people-centred.

> *We cannot continue to compromise all other social programs to fulfill the unrealistic goal of complete mental and physical well-being.*

A People-centred Report Card

I want each reader to be able to evaluate all proposals for health reform. To do this I have developed a *people-centred report card*. It is a convenient way to assess 10 aspects of health and health care that are fundamental to a people-first health system. The first six questions focus on the principles for moving beyond illness to health and wellness. The last four are examples of people-centred management. A rating of 1 indicates that the issue is not at all people-centred, and 5 that it is completely people-centred.

1. Individuality: Each person is unique. We must recognize our individual strengths and weaknesses and accept that there are no universal solutions to health issues. Does the issue support each person as a unique individual, or are people and providers asked to compromise their health goals to fit universal solutions?	**1 2 3 4 5**
2. Responsibility: To be healthy one must accept ownership for one's own journey to wellness. The true test is whether the stakeholders are accountable to the patient or to a third-party support group. For the issue, are people empowered and encouraged to take responsibility for their own health issues?	**1 2 3 4 5**
3. Informed: Healthy people are informed, and exercise their right to be the managers of their personal health. They demand information about legislation or treatment that can affect their well-being. Will the issue encourage people to inform themselves about what is possible for their personal health goals, regardless of whether it fits the current system?	**1 2 3 4 5**
4. Choice: There are always options in health and health care. Healthy people demand to know all their options in order to make appropriate choices. Does the issue give people all options or just those that fit the budget—can people exercise their choices with respect to services, providers, support groups, funding and management?	**1 2 3 4 5**
5. Quality: Healthy people personally define quality, and a people-centred system is based on the principle that no third party has the right to impose a definition of quality. People are encouraged personally to define and pursue the quality of care or service that meets their needs and expectations, and do not simply accept what the system is willing or able to provide. Does the issue allow people to pursue a personally defined quality of care or service?	**1 2 3 4 5**

6. Reality: Each person has time, energy, social, financial and environmental realities in his or her life. Healthy people use their strengths to overcome their weaknesses. The purpose of the publicly funded health safety net is to support people so they can overcome financial and accessibility realities. For the issue, are people able to define goals and pursue treatment based on personal realities, or does the government or provider determine reality based on the financial limits of the system?	**1 2 3 4 5**
7. People-centred definition of health: Health is a personally defined balance of mental, physical, spiritual and emotional well-being. Does the issue encourage people personally to define health, or are they expected to accept a universal definition?	**1 2 3 4 5**
8. The "yes, but…" factor: Various stakeholders claim to believe in a people–centred system but only if it supports their special interests. For example, we believe in people-centred health care but only if it fits within the *Canada Health Act*, or is not for profit, or is universal, or enhances the company's profit margin. For the issue, do the *buts* come before people-centred care?	**1 2 3 4 5**
9. People-centred working model: The patient is the nucleus of his or her personal health system, and all stakeholders are ultimately accountable to the patient. The current system is built on the belief that the *Canada Health Act* is the nucleus, and all stakeholders (including the patient) are accountable to the Act. Does the issue ensure account-ability to the patient?	**1 2 3 4 5**
10. One-tiered health care, or 32 million tiers: People-centred care means there are 32 million unique Canadians who ultimately have the choice of being responsible for and managing their own health. Unless and until there is one level of health, there can never be one-tiered health care. What society can strive for is a universally accessible level of support, but with people-centred care individuals have the choice of when, how or if they use the support. Does the issue support people-centred or system-centred care?	**1 2 3 4 5**

Total: _____

50 is completely people-centred, and 0 is completely system-centred.

All forms of support are possible in a people-centred system. The difference is the way they are implemented.

● ▲ ●

With the background, knowledge and tools provided in Part I, we're now ready to see exactly how we can bring in a people-centred system. Part II shows what reformed health care for Canadians would look like under the new *Canada Health and Wellness Act*: managing and funding the system, informing Canadians about health, and practical examples of health care.

SUMMARY—CHAPTER 5

- there is much work to be done if we want a system that will support the expectations of an informed and empowered people
- as we ponder the difference between "car" and "care", perhaps we should question whether health is the number one issue for Canadians
- a patient-centred report card can be a useful tool for evaluating all aspects of health care
- Canadians should set six realistic health goals for the nation:
  1. to define health and the principles of health and to make these the basic conditions for future health policy
  2. to inform, empower and support each individual as the potential manager of his or her own health
  3. to provide a universal level of support and implement it in such a way that it does not violate the first two goals
  4. to create an effective, efficient, accountable and sustainable health system that supports the health of the people
  5. to accept that change is inevitable, that information can change and that people are individuals, and never again to go 20 years without re-evaluating our health system, and
  6. to define the limits of what we as a nation are able and willing to do to support the health of the people, and to develop health policies that work within those limits

PART II

How We
Can Do It

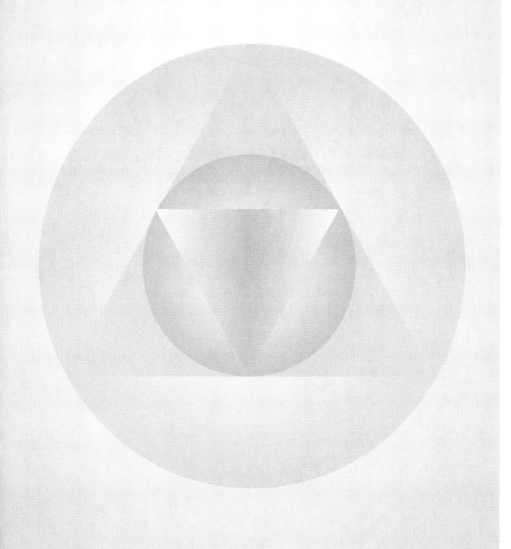

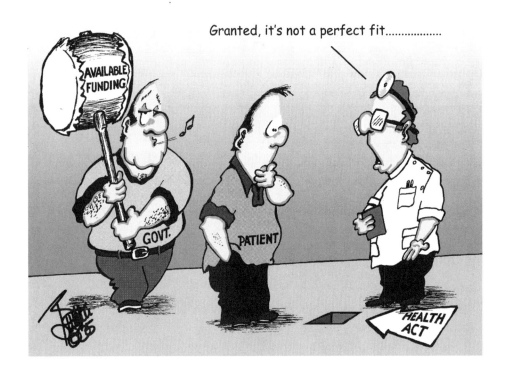

CHAPTER 6

The *Canada Health and Wellness Act*

The purpose of the health care system is to support the health of the people. The purpose of a Canada Health and Wellness Act *is to define the health rights of the people and protect them by law. It will ensure that the health of the people is not compromised by the agendas or objectives of the other stakeholders.*

I T IS TIME for some creative thinking. In Chapter 4 it was apparent that one of the greatest barriers to moving from disease to health is the lack of legislation that defines and protects the health rights and responsibilities for the individual. The fundamental legislation of the current system is the almost sacred *Canada Health Act*.

In my presentations and meetings on health reform, every political, business and professional group I have spoken to agrees that the system is a major part of the problem, and yet Canadians have had great difficulty conceiving any vision for a health system that does not centre on the existing Act.

We must develop a new Act, incorporating all that is good about what we have now and establishing the framework for a people-centred health system providing a more effective form of health support. This act I have called the *Canada Health and Wellness Act*.

The political conundrum

Most politicians have not thought about health care from a people-centred perspective—but to be fair, very few people have. Most politicians I have met are quite surprised that there is an alternative way of

Most politicians have not thought about health care from a people-centred perspective—but to be fair, very few people have.

looking at health care, one that addresses so many of the critical issues threatening the survival of the existing health system.

I believe that most politicians are honestly trying to make a difference and to act in the best interests of individual Canadian. They believe that the existing system is basically good and just needs a little tweaking. They believe this not because they understand the system or the *Canada Health Act*, or because they have invested years researching health care reform and understand or have ever thought about principles of health. They believe it because the leaders in their parties and the studies they are given say so. They have been told, and they believe, that the system is one-tiered (with a universal level of care), excellent and not-for-profit. Yet:

- our system is *not* one-tiered now—it never has been and it never will be
- our system does *not* provide excellence for all Canadians—it never has and it never will, and
- ours is *not* a not-for-profit system.

If you still believe that Canada has a not-for-profit system, consider the list of those who profit materially, personally, politically or professionally: the politician winning an election because of a health care platform that claims to be not for profit; the shareholder in a drug company; the health provider; the bureaucrat who makes an exorbitant salary as an advisor to all stakeholders; and the health care commission getting millions of dollars to do studies about why we should maintain the status quo.

Health care is an industry that is worth over $130 billion annually, and there have always been and always will be (and always should be) profits. The question is whether the profits should be more transparent, so the public can be more aware of what the profits are and make those receiving them accountable for their work.

Unfortunately there are also losses: those who lose every day and every minute because of a system that does not encourage accountability and alternatives. Too often this is the patient.

If politicians are going to continue to be the decision-makers on health issues, they owe it to their constituents and to all Canadians to study and understand what exists and the alternatives.

If politicians are going to continue to be the decision-makers on health issues, they owe it to their constituents and to all Canadians to study and understand what exists and the alternatives. They owe it to us to make informed decisions about the future of our health system. Unless each politician can find reasons to continue to support something other than a people-centred system, it is time for them to lobby for what is best for our health. Our political leaders can no longer say they are unaware of alternatives.

It is time for the political visionaries and entrepreneurs to put the health of the people ahead of what is politically correct or best for their party in the next election. It is time for all politicians to unite around the health needs of the people in 2005, and set out a path for our country to a true people-centred health system that meets those needs.

What can a *Canada Health and Wellness Act* do?

Designing a health Act is no easy task, but it may not be as difficult as we are led to believe because we have the basic framework in place. Chapter 5 outlined six national goals for a people-centred health system. Although these make theoretical and philosophical sense, many stakeholders have very different objectives and agendas, and many strongly want to maintain the status quo. There are businesses with corporate objectives and shareholder interests, political parties with very diverse philosophical and electoral agendas, provider groups with personal and professional interests, and 32 million unique individuals with specific personal goals. A national health Act must define the parameters within which each of these stakeholder groups will function.

I suggest most Canadians would agree that the overriding purpose of any health Act is not to support the shareholders of a company, a particular political party, a particular lobby group or a particular

> *...the purpose of the health Act is to make sure that our health is not compromised by the agendas or objectives of the other stakeholders.*

health philosophy. The purpose of the system is first to support the health of Canadians; thus the purpose of the health Act is to make sure that our health is not compromised by the agendas or objectives of the other stakeholders.

Political and lobby-group issues have played a major role in the design and implementation of the current Act. Questions such as whether the system should be for-profit or not-for-profit, privately or publicly operated, and universal or not, often dominate the dialogue. Each of these was a common catch phrase among political parties during the 2004 federal election. All these are issues about how the universal level of support is designed, but it is still just a support group like any other. Regardless of which side of any debate you support, it is important to make sure that it is accountable to an Act defining what health and wellness are in Canada.

Designing an Act around health rather than health around an Act

The first responsibility of a people-centred health Act will be to put into legislation the basic concepts that we have already outlined in Part I: a new definition of health (Chapter 2), the principles of health (Chapter 3) and the need for a people-centred model for health care (Chapter 4).

The second responsibility of the Act will be to allow all stakeholders to support health and be rewarded, as long as they support the basic concepts. To be part of a people-centred health system and to function within a proposed *Canada Health and Wellness Act*, a health care provider or support group must decide whether to be:

- for health or not for health
- for people first or not for people first
- for quality or not for quality
- for choice or not for choice
- for reality or not

- for informed and empowered patients or not, and
- for personal patient responsibility or not.

While the best decisions may appear to be obvious, it is worth remembering which decisions actually underlie the existing *Canada Health Act*. As we design a new health Act, we must constantly keep our goals in mind. Let us review a few of the conflicts that exist:

- It is no longer acceptable to compromise health goals to fit philosophical, financial or political beliefs.
- It is not acceptable to impose not-for-profit, public or universal agendas and in so doing force patients and providers to compromise their health goals.
- Not-for-profit is fine, but not if it eliminates choice, quality and personal decision-making power.
- Universality is good, but not if it compromises choice, quality, or responsibility.

In a system where health and people come first, the decision about whether to compromise is the right and responsibility of the individual.

But first, slay the dragon of one and two tiers

One of the greatest myths of the current *Canada Health Act* is that there is—or ever has been—a universal level of care. One-tiered health care is a political objective that has taken on a special meaning in Canada. Over my years of promoting health reform, I have found many forms of resistance to and negativity about changing the system. The greatest consternation appears at the suggestion that there could be a two-tiered health system, one for the rich and one for the poor.

But ever since the *Canada Health Act* came into force, various creative ways around the theoretical one-tier system have emerged and thrive today. In at least one case fully private health care is explicitly and legally provided: the program for members of the Canadian Forces and their families, at a cost of $90,000,000 annually.[37] Otherwise the most prevalent way around the one-tiered constraints is based on whom you know. Politicians, professional athletes, health care workers, doctors and their families and friends rarely have the same level of care or waiting lists as the general public.

The second way around the system is based on *what you know* and is often related to whom you know. When we are well-informed we can often get a different quality of care or service because we know to ask for it.

Another way around one-tier care is based on *power and influence*. Political, business and professional influence have created another level of care. A prominent medical malpractise lawyer once told me that he didn't understand what the problem was with access or waiting lists. He went on to explain that he has had a myriad of health problems, but the system was first class. When he needed an appointment his providers asked him what time would be convenient, and invariably saw him as quickly as he needed to be seen. Surgeries did not involve waiting lists or delays. The providers asked him when he wanted to be treated and which surgeon he preferred, and there were no delays or bumping of surgical times. He was astonished when he discovered what people who are not in his position have to live with.

Contrast this level of care to that received by Chris, the husband of a receptionist in our office, who had a serious problem with his oesophagus and was unable to swallow food. He required a complicated surgical procedure and he patiently went along with the system. His surgery was cancelled no fewer than seven times, but on the eighth time the family contacted influential people in the system and the surgery proceeded. He was unable to swallow solid foods for five months because he was unaware that the key to service is to play the who-you-know game.

> *The thought of people buying their way up waiting list is repulsive, yet it is no more repulsive than the current practise where people access treatment quicker because of whom or what they know.*

The thought of people buying their way up the waiting list is repulsive, yet it is no more repulsive than the current practise where people access treatment quicker because of whom or what they know.

When I first started to talk about health reform I was often branded a wealthy dentist trying to create a two-tiered health system, but that is the last thing on my mind. I had to find ways to get people to think differently. I have discovered that Canadians understand and can accept the idea of each person's uniqueness—that there are already 32 million personalized health systems in Canada, regardless of what any public-opinion poll says.

Once we get beyond this mental barrier and accept that we all have very different needs, and that the publicly funded health safety net is only one of many support options, then the challenge for the government becomes very different. It is no longer expected to be all things to all people.

In a people-centred system, the safety net will be the highest quality of care that the government is able and willing to provide for specified services, through a new *Canada Health and Wellness Act* that clearly defines the rules for all aspects of health and a health system. If any support system (public or private) is unable or unwilling to provide the service or quality of service that the individual needs, then it must be the right of the individual to pursue options.

Key Elements of The *Canada Health and Wellness Act*

1. *Clear direction for the new people-centred system*

The Act must provide for an all-inclusive definition of health, the principles of health, and a people-centred functioning model for health care.

2. *A basic universal level of support*

The Act must make sure that all people continue to have access to a basic level of care or support that will represent the minimum level of care all Canadians are entitled to.

3. *Recognize the diversity of Canadians*

The Act must recognize the needs of all Canadians. Each of us has a pathway to optimal health based on our needs, expectations and information. Whether we view ourselves as patients, clients, consumers or coaches, each of us should be able to pursue a personally defined level of health, health care and health support that must be protected in any future health Act.

4. *Third-party support groups cannot dictate the provider–patient relationship*

As we saw in chapter 1, it is unethical for a doctor to design his or her diagnosis and treatment plan around an insurance plan. It is the provider's responsibility to diagnose and present options based on what he or she feels is best for the health of the client.

Because a person has a particular social or financial status should not dictate the options a provider offers. These factors may affect the option the individual chooses to pursue, but that is the client's choice. The responsibility of the provider is to offer information about choices and to support the individual in creatively finding ways to achieve his or her health goals.

This is true in all of health care but this rule changes for those services covered under the existing *Canada Health Act*. If a particular service is considered to be medically necessary under the Act, then the provincial insurance plans dictate what treatment options physicians can be paid for. In health professions not controlled by the Act such as dentistry or optometry, this is unethical. Under the 1984 amendments to the *Canada Health Act*, it is an offence to provide a quality of service beyond that covered in the comprehensive clause of the act, and to be compensated for it. The fine for not abiding by the provincial plan can be many thousands of dollars.

Outside the current system it is a crime not to offer the options and it is assumed you would be rewarded for the service you provide. Inside the system it is a crime to offer the options and be rewarded for providing the service.

The proposed *Canada Health and Wellness Act* must eliminate this double standard of professional ethics.

5. *Encourage re-evaluation*

The Act must provide for regular re-evaluation of the various elements of the health system to ensure it remains responsive to the needs of the people.

An Action Plan for a People-Centred Health System

Designing a *Canada Health and Wellness Act* is a critical step in an action plan to move us to a people-centred health system. Without it, the best ideas for informing, empowering and supporting the individual will continue to be lost.

The idea of getting political parties among all levels of government to work together to create a non-partisan health and wellness Act seems an impossible dream, but I am convinced it is possible. Health should not be a political football. Health and health care needs do not change because one political party or another is elected. The parties can have philosophical differences about how they would use tax dollars and what percentage would go to health or education. But regardless of what party is in power, it is important to make sure that the patient is not held hostage if a government cannot or will not provide a service or quality of service. The Act must assure all individuals that they can become all they are capable of, and protect the health of the people from the limitations of the public system, not force us to be victims.

As an advocate for the patient, the Canadian Association for People-Centred Health will make this Act a priority in federal and provincial politics. If we can succeed, there will be no turning back on our journey to wellness.

Unless and until Canadians believe that the proposed system can be managed and funded properly and that the health of the people will benefit, there will be no momentum to change the existing system despite all its shortcomings. Assuming that the Act will be in place, we can now look in more detail at managing and funding a people-centred model—important parts of our overall action plan, and the subjects of the next two chapters.

SUMMARY—CHAPTER 6

In developing a people-centred health and wellness Act, we should remember that:

- the purpose of a system is to support the health of the people

- governments cannot manage health or health care: their role is to fund a defined level of care

- a *Canada Health and Wellness Act* must define health and the principles of health, and provide the guidelines for all stakeholders—the Act must support health, not create barriers to health

- health care is not one-tiered, nor has it ever been: there are 32 million personally defined health systems in Canada, one for each Canadian, and the challenge is to design a system that supports everyone

- a *Canada Health and Wellness Act* must incorporate five key elements:
  1. clear direction for the new people-centred system
  2. a basic universal level of support
  3. recognition of the diversity of Canadians
  4. assurance that third-party support groups cannot dictate the provider–patient relationship
  5. a system that encourages re-evaluation

- the *Canada Health and Wellness Act* is the first step in an action plan for reforming our health system

CHAPTER 7

Managing a People-Centred Health System

We need to turn the traditional management model upside down and keep responsibility, power and control as close to the patient as possible.

H OW THE PEOPLE-CENTRED health system is managed, and by whom, is critical to the success of the system. It is impossible to implement people-centred principles in a politically driven or doctor-centred system. This chapter describes three management models, and then examines the implications of people-centred management for the various levels of government.

> *It is impossible to implement people-centred principles in a politically driven or doctor-centred system.*

The Traditional Business Management Model

In the hierarchical industrial-age management model the boss, president, chief executive officer or doctor is always at the top. The support team, the workers, and finally the client or customer all fall somewhere under this figure of power and control. Graphically, this management model is a hierarchical pyramid with the control and power at the top. In a small or medium-sized business, for example, the pyramid of power might look like this:

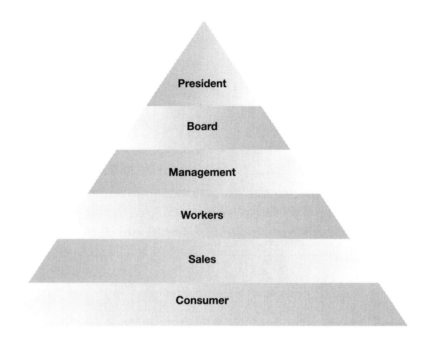

Fig. 7.1. Traditional business pyramid of power

The important point is that there are many levels of bureaucracy between the person with the power and the consumer who will use or buy the product or service.

The System-Centred Management Model

The current health system is designed around the *Canada Health Act.* A system-centred management model, it can be represented as a hierarchical pyramid of power with the Act at the top, providers in the middle and patients at the bottom. In this model, health goals are regularly compromised to fit the Act, rather than the system putting the needs of the patient first and adapting flexibly to our individual health goals.

The 50-year-old marathoner who cannot get a ceramic hip because the system covers replacements only for patients under a certain age, the doctor who recommends a prostate specific antigen (PSA) test for patients above a certain age because the system covers them only according to age, the multiple emergency appointments because the system will allow the doctor only to bill for one service at a time, and the rushed examinations because they must fit into either a $17, a $27 or a $47 fee range—all are examples of providers and patients compromising health goals to fit the system. The Act is non-negotiable and supports legislation that discourages and even fines a doctor if he or she receives payment for providing any of these options. If everyone can't have it, then no one can have it. This is the type of support the people receive in a system-centred management model controlled by system-centred legislation.

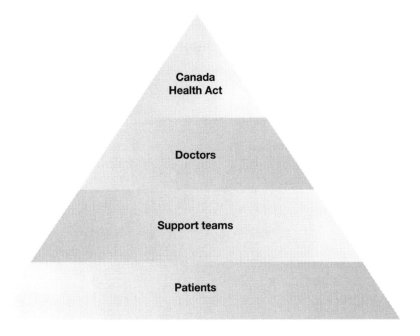

Fig 7.2. System-centred pyramid of power

Regardless of how much the doctor wants to empower and inform his or her patients, it is extremely difficult if the system is designed otherwise—doctors, health teams and patients are all subordinate to the Act. It is no surprise that informed people are challenging the system. It is very surprising to me that doctors, as the designated visionaries for health care, have been passively willing to compromise care to fit the system for so long.

Access to information is exposing the shortcomings of a health system that fails to put the health needs of the people first and promises to provide excellence and choice but is unable to do so.

After 20 years, this system-centred management model is suffering the same fate as many business or professional models. Access to information is exposing the shortcomings of a health system that fails to put the health needs of the people first and promises to provide excellence and choice but is unable to do so.

The Doctor-Centred Management Model

The traditional doctor's office follows a similar model. The doctor is all-powerful, and the nurses and support staff rarely challenge the authority or decisions of the doctor.

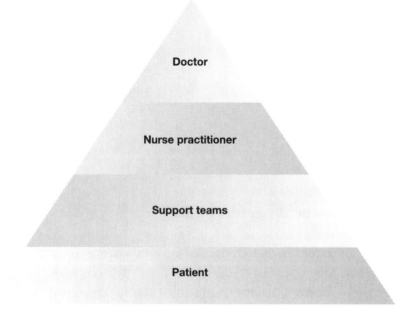

Fig. 7.3. Doctor-centred management model

In this model the patient is inferior to the doctor—rarely questioning why or what the doctor recommends. Most patients are reluctant to challenge the doctor, perhaps out of fear of being labelled a problem patient and likely being unable to find another doctor. Blind faith in the power figure worked well as long as people thought there was no alternative.

To this day many doctors are irritated by anyone, patient or team member alike, who challenges their authority. The doctor-centred model is all too familiar and is incongruent with

In this setting, too many health decisions are made without the consumer understanding why or what options are available.

the informing and empowering model we are trying to create. In this setting, too many health decisions are made without the consumer understanding why or what options are available.

When we were learning about patient-centred management in our dental office we were fortunate to find consultants to help us through this transition to a much more empowered team and patient. Suzanne Bekolay worked in our office for three months to assist us with communication and help our team (who were primarily focused on illness care and fixing problems) to become personal coaches and managers for an increasingly informed and responsible clientele. One lesson she emphasized was that we should never give people a solution until they recognize they have a problem. This simply means that with the exception of emergency care, you should never treat anything until the individual appreciates that he or she has a problem and should do something about it. Too often treatment plans are designed around what the provider values or believes is significant. The effective application of this idea, more than any other, has changed the way we work with our clients, and if implemented would have a dramatic effect on our health system.

The People-Centred Management Model

Our information age has created a very different environment. Knowledge is power, and over the past 20 years patients and providers have gained much better access to information about health relationships, to the point that most of us are able to manage our own health very effectively in many (and for some cases all) situations. This information-driven transition is creating a very different people-centred management model.

As people become more informed, they are refusing to be merely the submissive patients of powerful doctor-figures. They are demanding a much more active role as informed, empowered, thinking people who are able to research health issues, their symptoms and the possible causes. We can even make our own diagnoses. Our diagnoses are not always right, but right or wrong, what is significant is that many patients are very different from those arriving for medical appointments just 20 years ago.

> *People are demanding a much more active role as informed, empowered, thinking people who are able to research health issues, their symptoms and the possible causes.*

As informed clients of health care, we want to know our options, we regularly challenge the diagnoses, and even more often we challenge the treatment options that doctors recommend. We even challenge whether medical doctors are the best people to treat our particular problems. Canadians are choosing alternative medicine (homeopathy, naturopathy, acupuncture and counselling, for example) and getting several opinions before deciding how to deal with a health issue. We have turned the management and power triangle upside down.

> *If we choose to be managers of our own personal health systems, we must have the option to keep control and power in our own hands.*

As health consumers, we are starting to realize that to be healthy, we must accept responsibility for our own health. If we choose to be managers of our own personal health systems, we must have the option to keep control and power in our own hands. It is not only the informed patient who is leading this change. The coaches, support teams and various levels of management are also more informed and empowered, and are discovering that they have a significant role in supporting health care. They too are demanding change. The doctor-centred model is being attacked both internally and externally. The challenge is to help the doctors see that inverting the pyramid is in the best interests of everyone, including the doctors.

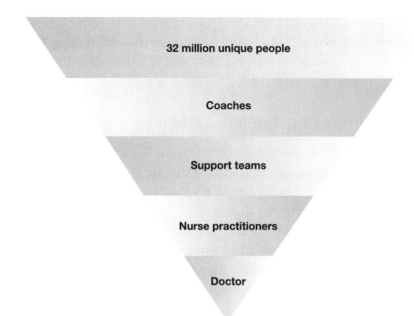

Fig. 7.4. People-centred pyramid of power and management model

In the people-centred model, the doctors fulfill a very different role as support persons for all the levels of support above them. They are still leaders and visionaries, but they must also be team leaders. Because of the expanded roles of patients, support-team members, nurses, nurse practitioners, client co-ordinators, social workers and many other alternative-health support groups, physicians are no longer just general practitioners who treat everything. They are able to assume the role of primary-care specialists who take over whenever the other levels of management are unable to fulfill the patients' needs. Doctors are the supports when all others fail.

The doctors in a people-centred model quickly begin to recognize that a high percentage of health clients are best served by team members other than themselves. They realize it is much more efficient, effective and sustainable if issues are managed by the first levels of the management pyramid. As the leaders and visionaries, they create systems that support this new approach. The doctor diagnoses and plans the treatment options if necessary, but delegating power and authority to the team member who is closest to the client—highest up on the inverted pyramid—is always the first choice. Again, this more effective and effi-cient use of providers' time and skills in a people-centred management model is possible only if we have a system that will recognize and com-pensate the team, or allow the people to compensate the team.

Personally Managing a Health System

The idea of personally managing our own health systems and being able to afford an acceptable level of care was an impossible dream 40 years ago. Now Canadians can have both, and are perfectly positioned to lead the way to fulfilling the dream. Two factors make this possible: we are committed as a nation to providing a universal level of support for the most expensive aspects of health care, and by world standards we have a highly educated public with an almost limitless ability to be informed and empowered in the future.

Questions from the public

In speaking with members of the public about personally managing their own health systems, I am often asked "What happens if I don't want to (or I can't) accept responsibility?"

In response, I suggest we consider two facts as we struggle with this new expectation. First, I have demonstrated in Chapter 3 that on average each of us is already managing our own health issues over 99% of the time without professional support. Second and more significantly, when we do get professional health-management advice, most of us choose to manage on our own anyway. Be it prescription drug compliance, exercise, nutri-tion counselling, smoking cessation, alcohol management, lifestyle or environmental changes or any of the treatment recommendations profes-sionals make, we take our health management into our own hands.

Questions from physicians

Doctors with whom I meet often express concern that if the doctor is not the primary contact person, urgent situations may be misdiag-nosed or delayed. The facts don't support this concern, and it may actually be the best reason for moving to people-centred management.

In Arnprior, Ontario where I live, as in most areas in the country, there is a perceived shortage of doctors. Several doctors are retiring, many doctors are not accepting new clients and most people are very concerned about not having a general practitioner. An October 2004 national survey showed that 60% of "all family physicians either limit the number of new patients they see or do not take new patients at all.... One-third of the specialists who responded to the survey indicated they could not see non-urgent cases referred from family physicians in less than three months."[38] In a nearby town there is only one practising physician for a population of 15,000 people, 10 fewer than the town needs.

We have already seen in Chapter 4 that only 31% of the billings of general and family physicians were for services that doctors alone can legally perform: 69% could have been provided by nurse practitioners, nurses and other health support staff or professionals.[39] If there is

Rather than have patients waiting weeks or months to see a doctor, why not have everyone immediately seen by a coach, so that people who truly need to see the doctor would be able to do so promptly?

a shortage of doctors, it makes sense to set up a practise model that screens clients and directs them as quickly as possible to the team members (other than the doctor) who can resolve their concerns. Rather than have patients waiting weeks or months to see a doctor, why not have everyone immediately seen by a coach, so that people who truly need to see the doctor would be able to do so promptly?

The resistance to general practitioners functioning more as specialists and working with an informed and empowered team is even more curious if we examine how other medical specialists work. In the existing professional model, patients must be referred to medical specialists by a general practitioner as a way of ensuring that specialists (who are in short supply) would use their time more effectively dealing with issues relevant to their expertise. Can properly trained and empowered nurses, nurse practitioners, consultants, client co-ordinators or coaches not begin to screen and even treat at least a portion of this 69% of the people who do not need to be on a waiting list for a doctor?

This could also be a start in dealing with the perceived shortage of specialists in our system. For example, it is common knowledge that one of the ways of dealing with the stress of too many patients is for family doctors to refer patients to specialists even though, if there were more time, many of their health issues could be treated by the primary-care physician. It would make sense if nurses, nurse practitioners and other health-support staff who are qualified to provide care were used more effectively to free up time for the family doctor. The doctor, in turn, could then take the time to provide services that are otherwise passed on to specialists.

I say "perceived" shortage of medical doctors because—in addition to the ineffective use of the doctors skills and support teams, as outlined in part one—I wonder if the shortage is actually a symptom of a system that ineffectively and inefficiently uses support and technology. I suggest that the doctor-shortage problem could be at least partly alleviated by implementing computerized record-keeping technology and hiring people at the administrative end so that nurses and nurse practitioners could be more effective and efficient in doing what they are trained and licensed to do. This would then allow the most expensive and highly trained people—the doctors—to focus on what only they can do: invasive procedures, diagnosis and treatment planning for the more complex health issues.

Using The People-Centred Management Model to Address Other Health Care Issues

The people-centred management model can play an invaluable role in clarifying how various stakeholders approach many of the continuing problems in health care. One example of this came up in discussions with my sister Linda, who is a registered nurse in a nursing home in the small town where I was raised. As the population ages, the demands on geriatric care services increase and complaints about the care our loved ones receive increase. As Linda told me, "we don't have the time, the staff, the support, the finances or the facilities to live up to the expectations of the families." Governments keep promising high-quality care so people expect it, but when the election is over these same politicians fail to follow through on their promises and the care-givers are left to cope with all the inadequacies of the system.

People-centred management can help people to move beyond political ideology and accept their appropriate roles. The first step is for people to begin to understand that the front line of support in any health system is always the individual or family. If people want affordable high-quality long-term care, they must appreciate that their role in geriatric care

…the front line of support in any health system is always the individual or family.

does not end the day they drop their loved ones off at the home. Professional support is still the last line of support, and unless people are willing to pay for this costly professional care, they must be prepared to continue to visit and be the first line support on all matters except those that only the trained professional can provide. The system was not designed to pay for comprehensive, high-quality chronic care, and politicians must stop making promises they cannot fulfill.

This type of delegation of responsibility back to the individual or family is very unpopular politically. No politicians win votes when they tell the electorate that they are expected to do more, but it is essential for the survival of the system and more importantly for the care of our aging population. Once again people must accept that no third party (regardless of what a politician running for office promises) can be all things to all people. If people want high quality, there are roles for the individual and the family that the current system is ignoring and trying to pass on to already overburdened health workers. Politicians must either pay for the facilities and the professional people to care for our loved ones properly, or tell voters the truth. This is another reason why health care can no longer be a political football for politicians during elections.

Governments' roles in a people-centred system

The existing model for governing is centralized by design, and keeps the power and control in the hands of the higher levels of government—the federal and provincial governments much more so than the municipal levels. Graphically, the traditional government management model can be represented as a pyramid of power:

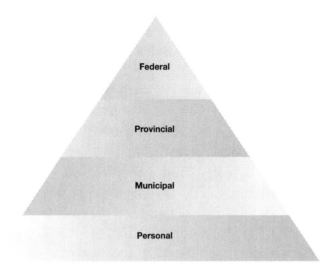

Fig. 7.5. Traditional government management model

If the roles of governments are to develop policies that inform, empower and support our health through a new *Canada Health and Wellness Act*, there is a need for a very different hierarchy. By inverting the government model, we have an empowered person being supported by all other levels of government—a people-centred government management model:

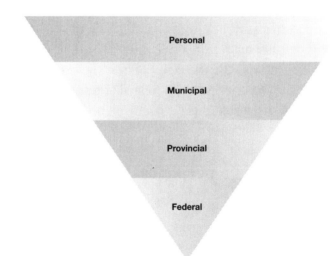

Fig. 7.6. People-centred government management model

With this people-centred model in mind, let's consider each level of government.

The personal level

As we make the transition to a people-centred management model, we'll start to recognize a personal level of government (or empowerment, if you prefer). It is actually the most important level of governance because it empowers all 32 million Canadians to manage most of our own health issues. The personal level is the first line of control, and it is only when this level fails to cope with health issues that the other levels of support come into play.

In the existing system, too many people believe they are victims and that life decisions are beyond their control. This feeling of being victimized is the result of a system that is parental in nature. In a people-centred management model individuals must have options and be encouraged to set their health goals and make conscious decisions about their lives and the way they live.

The individual's roles in governing this personal level of health are:

- to define health and a personally relevant balance of mental, physical, spiritual and emotional well-being
- to embrace a personal definition of health and the six principles of health, and
- to be the visionary for his or her own personal health.

By recognizing personal support as the most powerful level, and by encouraging personal responsibility, we will immediately affect the inefficiencies of the system. This is the practical application of the people-centred model. When people stop depending on others, they begin to find health solutions through self-management, being informed, accepting responsibility, making choices, defining quality, and using all the resources and support avail-

If even a small percentage of the population can accept a bigger role in self-governing, this will greatly affect a system that is trying to cope with an aging and increasingly ill population.

able without ever involving the professional medical care-givers. If even a small percentage of the population can accept a bigger role in self-governing, this will greatly affect a system that is trying to cope with an aging and increasingly ill population.

When I make the case for expecting increased responsibility, a common comment from providers and patients is that most people will not or are not capable of taking on increased responsibility. I have two responses. First, I stress that people manage their health over 99% of the time and often ignore the management advice they get for the remaining 1%. Second, I recognize that many or most people will continue as they are now and accept whatever the system is willing to give them, but I disagree that most people are incapable of taking responsibility. If we begin to give people the information they need to make decisions and give them options, nearly everyone (with his or her personal friends, coaches and family) is more than capable. In fact, most will demand the right to make choices and, therefore, assume responsibility on health issues.

To begin the transition to a patient-centred system, patient-centred government (like management) must be an option. This means that the most powerful aspect of governing health must rest with the individual person, if he or she chooses. The difference is that the choice for all health matters is not legislated but is personal.

Some believe that this type of empowerment will destroy the system, but again we must ask whether the role of the system is to treat illness or support health. If it is to support health then we have to search for a hierarchy of government that supports the six principles of health.

Municipal (Community) government

The next level of government in our people-centred model is municipal government. As we evolve to a wholistic health system rather than just treating illness, it becomes apparent that the municipality and its resources have the most direct effect on the quality of our daily lives. Although Canadians invest hours debating federal and provincial politics, the more personally relevant politics of the municipality—the libraries, hockey rinks, roads, transit systems, water, sewage, recreational facilities, church groups, municipal bylaws and social programs—influence our well-being most immediately. If we and our personal support network cannot provide the basic needs for our well-being, then our community is the next line of defence.

Municipal governments deal with health issues, but are focused less on medical or physical health and more on social and environmental health. I don't know of any research that has studied how many health issues could be dealt with or eliminated completely if the power of the community and personal relationships were recognized and empowered. If we assume that the need for attention and personal interaction accounts for many of the 69% of medical visits that do not require the doctor's expertise, a caring community would most likely be best able to cope with a percentage of the personal, intangible aspects of our well-being that can't be measured at other levels of government. The ability of the community to know each of us as a unique person and to personalize our support is perhaps its greatest strength. After personal management, it is the next choice for support, wherever and whenever possible.

Provincial and territorial government

The primary role of provincial and territorial governments in our current health system is to administer the finances for the publicly funded, universal health safety net as directed by national policy—the most expensive, professionally dominated portion of health support. This level of government is generally responsible for public institutions such as hospitals, and the provinces and territories must work with federal health programs to make sure that all levels of health support, including professional and community health care, receive appropriate public funding for the needs of the people in their jurisdictions. The provincial and territorial governments set and collect their own taxes, which they use (together with contributions from the federal government) to finance their health care systems.

Perhaps the greatest challenge for provincial and territorial governments in a people-centred model will be to develop policies and strategies for the public health safety net that support the personal and community levels of government, but do not violate the principles of health. It is difficult to imagine how they will implement sup-

> *It is impossible simply to modify the existing system and achieve the desired support network. There must be real change.*

port programs while still respecting the right of each of us to accept responsibility and ownership, to be informed, to make choices, to define quality care and to do all this based on the realities in our own lives. In particular, how they handle funding and distribute health care information needs reforming—areas that we explore in the next two chapters. It is this level of management that exemplifies the need to change the way we look at things and develop a people-first system. It is impossible simply to modify the existing system and achieve the desired support network. There must be real change.

The federal government

The control of and responsibility for the national health system ultimately rests in the hands of the people, but taking national interests into account, the federal government is the only level that can create the legislation to ensure that every Canadian's health rights are respected and honoured by all levels of government.

The proposed *Canada Health and Wellness Act* is the first essential piece of legislation required to establish a people-centred model, but it can come about only if the federal government is on side. To this end, the federal government has six clear responsibilities:

1. *legislation:* to work with all stakeholders to define "health", define the principles of health, and put forward a *Canadian Health and Wellness Act* that would enable and accelerate the transition to a people-centred system.
2. *a seamless safety net:* in co-operation with the other levels of government, ensure that all levels work together to provide a seamless health safety net for all Canadians. In the past, the federal government has been the manager of the health system, but in a people-centred model this must change.
3. *stable management:* to set up a management structure ensuring long-term continuity and stability for the system. Changing management every four years at election time, or every two or

three years when the prime minister shuffles the cabinet, creates chaos in health care. Canada's health policy is suffering because of political instability, party politics and a continuing preoccupation with what promises might win an election.

4. *national funding model:* to collect and distribute the portion of the financial support for the universal health safety net that the provincial governments are unable to provide. The collection of funds for health care through various forms of taxation is well-established in legislation. The greatest challenge to the federal government is to find a mechanism for distributing provincial and federal funds that will empower each individual. We need to develop a national funding model where the buck stops with the individual, where the individual is at the centre of a personal health system, and a model in which providers and support groups are accountable to the individual for material reward.

5. *limits to support:* to work with providers, patients and support groups to clearly define the limits of support for the universal health safety net. Health care is a continuum and must be free to change and grow as our values change and grow. In a perfect world every one of us would have unlimited access to excellence in care, but this is not a perfect world.

The costs of health support are potentially limitless, and could consume every penny of tax revenue. There are limits to what the tax payer is able to provide, but these have never been defined. The result has been nearly uncontrolled deficit financing, and even this has its limits. Canadians say that health care is their number-one issue, but no one expects us to abandon all other social programs to support health. The federal and provincial governments must work together to establish clear guidelines for the percentage of tax dollars that can be invested in health, and then live within these guidelines.

If the federal government is unable to continue its level of support because of external or internal factors, the solution is not another waiting list or deficit financing. When this happens, the responsibility moves up to the next level. The goals of the patient could remain the same but the level of support and who provides it would change. If all levels of support or government are unable to address the patient's needs, it ultimately falls to the individual patient. If the patient is unable to find ways to achieve his or her goals, then either the goals must change or the patient must accept the universal level of care. This may seem harsh to mant Canadians, but it is much more democratic than the present model. Currently, if the federal government can't support a health need then we must all wait until the government decides it can.

6. *rewarding providers:* to establish a national plan for rewarding providers, there must be a list of comprehensive services covered in the health safety net. The federal government must work with providers to determine reasonable fees for services covered by the universal support system, and it must go into much more detail than what exists now. This list must define the limitations of what is covered, how long the patient should expect to wait for a procedure, when and where it will be provided, who can provide it and who will pay for it. It is then essential that all this information be available to patients and providers: information about all health services regardless of whether they are universal or personal, public or private, for-profit or not-for-profit. This is the information we need to be the managers for our own personal health systems.

As part of the plan, the list of services must also define what quality of service is covered. It is not sufficient to say examinations or hips or counselling are covered. Clearly defining the acceptable range of intangible services is a critical issue in moving to a system that supports the principles of health and functions within the financial limits of the system. The stakeholders must have access to all details of what is covered for each procedure, so they can evaluate a reasonable reward for what goes beyond the basic range.

We Need a Canadian Health Care Commission

At presentations over the past years, I have discovered from audiences that there is rapidly growing support for the idea that governments should no longer manage and administer health care. It is impossible to run a health system where the ministers of health are appointed for

It is impossible to run a health system where the ministers of health are appointed for political reasons and often have little or no background in health.

political reasons and often have little or no background in health. After each cabinet shuffle there is an extended period during which leadership is absent. This is generally followed by a change in policy. Even worse, each time there is a change in government there can be drastic changes in policy based on political ideology, egos, party policy or public opinion polls. The result is a system that is in constant turmoil and is too often in chaos.

The governments should finance the publicly funded and administered health safety-net insurance plan through tax revenue, but the system should be managed and administered by an independent, nonpolitical health care commission to which all health support groups are accountable. It should include members from all stakeholders in the business of health care. If a support group or government policy infringes on the principles of the *Canada Health and Wellness Act* or patient–provider relationships, there must be a non-partisan regulatory board with the power to intervene. This commission would:

- be an advocate for patients to ensure that support groups (including government) remain accountable to the patient, and that the system and stakeholders are patient-centred in word and action
- enforce the *Canada Health and Wellness Act* and make sure that providers and consumers fulfill their rights and responsibilities, and
- ensure that the support groups do not create barriers to the relationship between providers and patients.

People-centred management means we will have to look at creative new ways of funding our people-centred system, a major transition in thinking that is the focus of the next chapter.

SUMMARY—CHAPTER 7

The transition to a people-centred management model means that:

- the inverted hierarchical pyramid will involve many adjustments in how providers and organizations relate to one another and how they manage issues

- responsibility, power and control will be kept as close to the patient as possible and will empower all levels of support to fulfill their roles

- there are many more options. Just because a level of government cannot achieve something does not mean it is unachievable: it simply means we must look for different options. It is unacceptable to make someone wait a year for a hip replacement in Ontario and only three weeks in Quebec, simply because the governments' financial abilities differ or their priorities happen to be different.

- the use of teams will increase. There will be a transition from a doctor- or system-centred to a people-centred management model that is supported by a health team—the first point of contact is not necessarily the doctor. Having the doctor as the last line of defence instead of the first makes sense. The doctor will no longer try to be all things to all people. Doctors will be part of the team, but their roles will change.

- there is a clear need for a non-partisan, independent commission that ultimately controls and manages all stakeholders, including the various levels of government. The commission is accountable to the *Canada Health and Wellness Act*.

CHAPTER 8

Funding a People-Centred Health System

If Canadians were to stop funding all other social programs (including education) and invest every tax dollar in the current illness system, everyone would still get sick and die. We must define the limits of public support. We must find ways to support health, not just treat illness.

IN MY PRESENTATIONS on the people-centred health system proposal, questions about how we will fund it always come up. The answer is simple: any way we want, provided it is implemented in such a way that it supports the definition and the six principles of health. It is not acceptable to continue to throw a major portion of our national and provincial revenues into health without a clear vision of what health is or what our goals are. Illness care is a bottomless financial pit and it is time to deal with this.

Canadians seem to think they can do no wrong by putting money into illness care. However, if we compromise other worthy issues such as education, nutrition, agriculture, the environment and many other programs simply to treat more illness, we are cutting off our nose to spite our face. If we begin to look at things in a wholistic way, then we recognize that each of these is an important

To be a healthy or well nation we must accept that all the money in the world will extend the inevitable by only a few years, and possibly the psychological effects of saving and rescuing may be shortening the quality of life we enjoy.

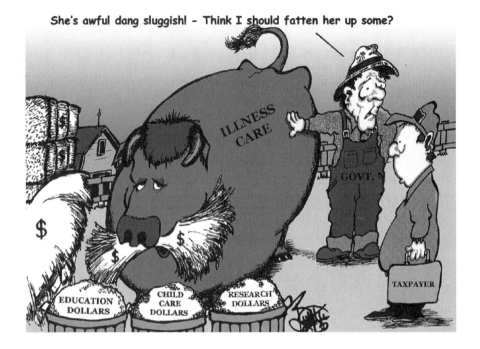

piece of the health puzzle. Once again we are forced to decide where to draw the line between health and illness.

Perhaps the most important of the six principles is finally to accept reality. To be a healthy or well nation we must accept that all the money in the world will extend the inevitable by only a few years, and possibly the psychological effects of saving and rescuing may be shortening the quality of life we enjoy. With these thoughts in mind, let's now search for the criteria for a funding mechanism that informs, empowers and supports each person as the manager of his or her personal well-being.

Empowering the Individual

The buck stops where the power is. If the government controls the health purse strings, it controls health care. What we need instead is a model for funding where the buck clearly stops with the only person who can determine that a service has met his or her needs and expectations: the patient.

The funding system and the way it is implemented will make or break the next-generation health system. We can never have a patient-centred system if we continue to use a politically motivated and controlled funding system that ignores the role of each individual. People must be the financial managers of their own personal health.

We can never have a patient-centred system if we continue to use a politically motivated and controlled funding system that ignores the role of each individual.

Purchasing Access to Care?

One of the principles of the people-centred model is that the individual should be able to explore all options for care, materials or services, and to obtain these options. *It is essential to understand that this does not mean that any individual can buy access to care.*

The people-centred model

It is essential to understand that this does not mean that any individual can buy access to care.

recognizes that there are many reasons other than who is first on the waiting list to determine who should have access to care. It also asserts that it is impossible to design legislation, write laws or appoint bureaucracies that are capable of determining fair and reasonable access priorities. The model must go beyond the tangible and material basis for access to recognize that in a situation with limited numbers of doctors and access to doctors, each life is valued. Money should not be the vehicle for quicker access to care, nor should access be defined as one set of rules for the wealthy and another for the poor.

Politically, this can be construed as the very unpopular practise where doctors help certain people jump the queue. But the reality is that health care providers are often the only people who are able to resolve access issues in a fair and humane way. For example, consider the quandary of the physician scheduling a heart transplant. A 12-year-old urgently needs a new heart, while the 70-year-old who is first on the waiting list has already had one transplant, continues to smoke and drink, and refuses to exercise or follow a rehabilitation plan.

Issues like this are problems that the current system cannot manage. Health professionals must make many difficult decisions about what, when, where and for whom health services are provided, and the funding system must support these decisions.

Purchasing Options, Not Access

The funding system must be designed to recognize our individual right to information, choice and quality. When we get to the head of the access line, the service to be provided should be at the discretion of the individual and his or her providers, advisors and support groups. Just as informed consent is a legally supported right, each of us has a right to have all our options explained and each of us—with the help of our providers—will determine which option best meets our personal situation.

The health safety net guarantees all of us access to a defined universal quality of care, but as we discussed in the previous chapter there are limits, and it does not necessarily provide universal excellence. In a people-centred system where the first priority is each individual's health, the patient and his or her health advisors must be empowered to determine how they use the limited publicly funded services. The individual, not the system, must determine whether he or she is able to supplement the universal level of care to achieve a more personally relevant level of care or quality of service—whether the price is time, energy, finances, environmental or social considerations.

> *The individual, not the system, must determine whether he or she is able to supplement the universal level of care to achieve a more personally relevant level of care or quality of service—whether the price is time, energy, finances, environmental or social considerations.*

Payment Systems

Financial reward for health services is the subject of much debate in Canada. On the one hand, true socialists believe that health care should be free for all and that doctors should be employees of the state and paid as such. On the other, true capitalists believe that free enterprise is the only answer and competition and a free market will result in the highest quality.

Is it possible to have a health care reward system based on the principles of health rather than whether it is for-profit or not-for-profit, public or private, or individual or universal? I suggest that three main options present themselves: fees for services, outcome-based rewards, and patient-centred rewards. Any of these can work, provided it supports the principles of health.

Fees for services

Before socialized health care, the most common way for providers to be rewarded was by fees for services. The patient received services from a doctor, was billed a fee for the service provided, and paid the bill with money, services, chickens, pigs or anything the patient had to trade.

This system survived for hundreds of years, based on one fundamental principle: the patient was paying the doctor for the service. The doctor was accountable to the patient, and therefore the system was patient-centred. The doctor's reward was based on whether the patient's needs were met—a built-in quality-control mechanism. There was no written fee guide, but people talked about costs and there was a general understanding of what fees were acceptable for a particular service. The provider and patient usually lived in close proximity as members of the same community, so the fees could vary depending on the ability of the individual to pay. In the absence of social support (beyond that offered by churches, synagogues and mosques), the community pulled together when someone was in need, and often the doctors donated their services as acts of charity.

Many Canadians are not aware that the current financial reward system under the *Canada Health Act* is based primarily on a fee for service. Each service covered under the Act has an accepted fee associated with it, as set out in a fee guide. This guide was created by political and professional committees and is reviewed and updated regularly. If a service qualifies for reimbursement by the system, the provider submits a code electronically for the services provided and at the end of the month receives a cheque.

For any fee-for-service system to work, the services must be precisely defined and the provider must be accountable to an informed consumer to be paid. This means that the patient, provider, and any support group financing the care must have a shared understanding about what should be included in the service to qualify to be paid.

Although there are always differences in the skills of the providers and the needs of certain patients, the current system works extremely well for many of the tangible, measurable aspects of care. For instance, there is a fee for setting an arm with a cast. The cast is a tangible item, and when the cast is applied both the patient and the provider can agree that the obligations of the service are fulfilled. There is little dispute that payment is justified. The problem is that most health issues are not as easily measured and managed as a cast.

As health care issues become more complex, the reward system under the current *Canada Health Act* and the way it is implemented present several disadvantages:

- *lack of accountability to the patient:* unlike the barter-style health care of the past where the doctor was directly accountable to the patient, the patient has been removed from the reward process. Patients do not pay the provider for the service. In fact they most often do not know what the provider bills the system for and what the expectations are for a particular service.
- *the patient is no longer involved in quality control:* the reward process is based on whether something is done to the patient, but since the patient does not give approval for the bill or even see the bill, there is no opportunity for him or her to express satisfaction or dissatisfaction with the service provided.
- *uniform fees don't acknowledge special skills:* the reward system is too often based on the unrealistic premise that all providers and all patients are the same, and the fee levels don't reflect the quality, time or difficulty involved in providing the service. We have one fee for an examination or hip replacement surgery or maternity care, even though each person is a unique individual and the abilities of the provider are unique.

- *inability to reward the intangibles:* as we become better informed we are looking for more than the tangible aspects of health care. We are looking for the care in health care: intangibles such as listening, communication, empathy and affection, the hands-on people skills that often determine whether we are satisfied with our care or not. These intangibles are not measurable by anyone but the patient, so how can a system that isolates the patient from the reward process recognize and reward this type of service? As a result the intangibles are becoming less and less a part of the system, and those providers who do take the time to provide them are being penalized because they spend more time with each patient for the same fee.
- *restricts the type of care:* as financial constraints are forcing provincial governments to cut services, more people are recognizing that the system is not universal and is only directed at people with certain illnesses who believe that western medicine is the treatment of choice. The Ontario government recently cut eye examinations and chiropractic services— prime examples of political decisions for political reasons. They had to cut something and they chose the services with the least political clout.

In a people-centred system there must be the option of rewarding the intangible aspects of care. For example, when my wife Betsy had a very difficult 32-hour labour and delivery with our first daughter, Amy, our doctor slept at the hospital, investing long hours to support us through this crisis. Our doctor did not have to do this nor does the system say he should, but he went above and beyond the call of duty and delivered a perfect baby girl and a healthy mother. No one could place a value on that level of care.

I wanted to do something in return for his exceptional care, but the system would not allow it. I was shocked to find that whether a doctor invests 32 hours or 32 minutes in a delivery, the financial reward is the same. He could actually have been fined for accepting a fee over and above what the *Canada Health Act* defines for deliveries.

Does this system encourage a doctor to pursue excellence, or does it encourage—and even force—the health care system into mediocrity? After 20 years' experience under the current health act, the results are ten-minute medical appointments, doctors checking their watches if the patient starts to talk too much, and most importantly a very frustrated medical community that wants to be able to offer the intangibles of health care but are rewarded for how many people they see and not how well they take care of them. We must develop a system that puts an end to this type of insanity.

Outcome-based rewards

Theoretically, under an outcome-based reward system, the doctor is rewarded for successfully achieving a desided outcome instead of being paid for providing a specific treatment. An example of outcome-based reward is *capitation* or *payment per person*.

As I am writing this chapter, the Ontario government is attempting to introduce a new payment-per-person reward system. In this proposal, doctors are to be paid $102 per person per year to provide primary health care for their clients. They are not paid for what they do. They are paid per person whether they do a lot or nothing. Many providers look at this as an opportunity to provide quality care and stop the rat race of fee-for-service care. In the United States, health maintenance organizations (HMOs) use a form of payment per person, except that they are privately funded. But is the publicly funded capitation model going to be any different?

As with other systems, outcome-based rewards have both advantages and disadvantages. On the positive side:

- The model provides a level of care for everyone based on the same principles as all insurance plans. The insured pays premiums knowing that if catastrophic illness or emergencies arise, everyone will share in the costs. Theoretically the doctor is paid to care for his patients as a group. This sounds nice in theory, but to generate enough income at $102 per patient, the doctor must rely on the fact that a small percentage of the people will use the services. (It seems curious to me that the annual cost of taking care of me or my loved ones is roughly 1.5 times the cost of an emergency visit from my plumber— somehow $102 suggests that my doctor will likely not be able to provide his or her best and finest for an increasingly informed and demanding clientele.)

- It is probably the easiest for the government to manage. The measurement is per person, and therefore is much less complicated than the fee-for-service system.

The outcome-based reward system is useful in certain circumstances and should be considered as a payment option, but until there is a way of keeping the patient at the centre it will be impossible to manage and achieve the goals of the informed patient.

Unless it is implemented properly, there are many disadvantages:

- There is no incentive to hire team members to enhance the quality of care. Doctors are paid a set amount per person, whether they have all kinds of support staff or work alone. There is no incentive to invest in excellence.
- Too often there is no definition of what the patient should receive or the provider should provide. This could easily be remedied, but the system must still give options for how people can receive services or quality of care above and beyond those covered by the per-person rate.
- Doctors are discouraged from accepting chronically ill patients. They are rewarded the same whether they do anything or not.
- There is no incentive to inform and empower the patient because the provider who does the least for the most people is rewarded the most.
- Patients are not involved in the remuneration process; in fact doctors are rewarded more depending on how many patients they don't see.
- Quality is arbitrary, and is not necessarily based on fulfilling the needs of the patient. Reward is based on doing as little as possible with the greatest number of people. In a perfect world with a surplus of doctors competing for clients and the

quality could be controlled, but in a system that is under-serviced with patients deemed lucky even to have a doctor, the option of going to another doctor if needs are not met is unrealistic.

This type of system has been tried throughout the world under various different names and programs, but it always comes back to this fact: unless the patient is at the centre of the model, there is no accountability and it becomes a game for those who want to play the system and make the most money for the least amount of time and energy invested.

Patient-centred rewards

Is there an option that takes the best of both models and truly addresses the needs of the individual? What is an ideal people-centred rewards system and what must it do?

- It must pay for a universal level of support for the highest possible quality of care it can afford, and allow people to identify all options and pursue what is best for them whether the coverage is universal or not.
- It must make sure that the doctor is ultimately accountable to the patient.
- It must not only reward providers for what they do (the tangibles), but also for how they provide the services (the intangibles).
- It must ensure that all people—regardless of material wealth—have equal access to a defined level of health services.
- It must encourage providers to develop efficient and effective support teams.
- It must support the people-centred principles of health.

No reward scheme can be successful if it ignores the needs of the provider. An effective people-centred reward system recognizes the needs of all stakeholders, not just the patient. The ultimate goal for any provider is to be rewarded financially, mentally, spiritually and personally, and most importantly with satisfied patients.

To be people-centred, the system must put the individual patient in the centre of the reward process. The reward is determined directly between the informed patient and the provider team, who clearly understand what their roles are. Together they clarify the patient's goals and develop a list of options to achieve the goals. Then they explore which options are available and realistic, and the patient chooses the most suitable option. Together they find ways to achieve the option that the patient has chosen. In effect, the patient determines the provider's reward. This flexible approach means that all third-party payment systems are possible, so long as they are not implemented in any way that violates the principles of health for the patient.

Such a system takes more work and involves a team approach, but for the provider the satisfaction of defining and fulfilling the needs of the patient and dealing directly with the patient is worth it. The other advantage is that the patient becomes the quality-control officer.

Designing A People-Centred Funding System that Supports Health

Internationally, the most common form of health care funding is a combination of public and private funding, such as in Sweden and in the United Kingdom. Canada is the only member of the Organization for Economic Co-operation and Development "that outlaws privately funded purchases of core services. Every other OECD country has some form of user-pay, private provision of health care."[40] We must seek ways to redesign the funding so that it supports our health regardless of how much funding is available.

There are many possible funding options, and most could work in a people-centred system. The difference is that they must be implemented in such a way that they support the goals outlined in Chapter 5.

For the purposes of this discussion I will highlight some of the reasons for reconsidering the concept of individual health savings accounts for at least a portion of health care funding.

What is a Publicly Funded Individual Health Savings Account?

Several countries and many corporations have introduced a very practical concept for having the buck stop with the patient—health savings accounts, or HSAs. Also known as medical savings accounts (MSAs), they have had varying degrees of success throughout the world, depending on the system in which they are implemented. Although HSAs have been advocated in Canada before, the concept was never accepted because it did not fit in a politically or provider-centred system. However, HSA's do fit in a system designed to inform and empower the individual.

To be effective the HSA incorporates three elements: a basic health savings account, a deductible account that comes into effect after the basic account is used up, and an insurance plan for health catastrophes.

1. *The basic health savings account: how it works*

The first element of each HSA is a basic account that is managed by the insured person. It is a publicly funded bank account that each Canadian would have for minor health expenses such as regular office visits, drugs and any minor services that the insurer agrees qualify (the insurer is the provincial or federal government or the manager of the public health funds).

The insurer would determine the amount that each Canadian would have in his or her account each year, and it would operate similarly to a debit card. Each account has a personal identification number (PIN) that would allow the patient to approve a withdrawal from the account. Similarly, each provider would have a PIN, and each service or procedure would have a numerical code.

Let's illustrate how the account works during Bob's visit to a doctor for a medical examination. Bob calls for an appointment at the office of his choice. He arrives and gives his personal identification number. His PIN confirms that he is a Canadian and that he's currently covered for health services. He is fully aware that he will be investing money from his personal health savings account—his own money, since it comes from his taxes. At this point Bob would want to understand his options for the examination and choose what form of examination would best fulfill his health needs. A member of the health team would then explain the options and the related costs and Bob would decide how to proceed. By having information about what the examination should cover, he is the quality-control officer for his personal health system.

After his examination by the doctor, the secretary presents the bill to Bob. The secretary enters the provider's number in the office computer, together with the code for the services performed. This confirms whether the office is eligible to receive payment for the services provided. Bob then goes through the same steps as for a debit card transaction: he approves the services he received for the fee, enters his PIN, and his account is debited electronically by the amount of the bill.

This example indicates how the health savings account involves all six of the principles of the people-centred model. The patient must be treated as a unique individual and not just another number. He becomes an active participant in the business process because he must

Simply by having the individual pay for the service encourages both the insured patient and his provider to be informed, accept responsibility, make choices and define the quality of the service.

approve the bill and confirm that the services were provided and that he received the expected outcome. Simply by having the individual pay for the service encourages both the insured patient and his provider to be informed, accept responsibility, make choices and define the quality of the service. At the same time, the insured patient's paying from his own health account acts as a deterrent to many of the perverse incentives of the current system that I noted in Chapter 1.

Unused balances in a basic account

At the end of the year, when the health account is about to be refilled with the next year's full amount, some people may have an unused balance. Should Canadians be allowed to transfer part or all of an unused balance from one year to the next? In my opinion, yes. For example, unused balances over a predetermined amount could be used to pay for health services whether or not they are included in the list of comprehensive services covered by the basic account. It may also be worth considering allowing these balances to be used to support other family members or an alternative quality of care for a catastrophic health event, or for covering the deductible amount in a deductible account, discussed below. The creativity of the stakeholders will ultimately determine the most effective use for these funds, but this is an issue that will have to be clarified.

2. *The deductible account*

The second level of the health savings account system is a deductible account, which would come into effect after the basic account is exhausted and before catastrophe insurance takes effect.

A deductible is essential in implementing a people-centred funding system. Although at first glance this may seem unfair to those who are financially disadvantaged, there are sound reasons why a deductible would benefit the financially compromised Canadian system. Provisions can readily be made that would support those who are unable to manage the additional costs.

The deductible is an incentive for us to think about how we use our health savings account. Some people may feel that all we are doing is introducing another tax and another level of bureaucracy. For others who believe there is no financial crisis and no misuse or abuse of the system, and those who are willing to turn over their health care to an insurer, these changes seem redundant.

One of the greatest threats to the future financial sustainability of the current system, however, is that many Canadians view health care as free—that somehow, because we are Canadian, we have an inherent right to health care and no matter how much we use or abuse this right, it will always be there when we need it. Telling us it is not so does not work. When financial reward is determined by how much a doctor, hospital, patient or administrator uses the system, there is a built-in incentive to overuse or misuse the system. Giving each of us a health savings account and making each of us a part of the process will help, but there is nothing like having to reach into our own pockets and spend some of our hard-earned dollars to drive home the fact that health funding is not limitless. It will also help people to understand that

Giving each of us a health savings account and making each of us a part of the process will help, but there is nothing like having to reach into our own pockets and spend some of our hard-earned dollars to drive home the fact that health funding is not limitless.

the reason Grandmother is waiting two years for her hip replacement is because people who abuse the system made seven trips to the emergency room for a cold that could have been handled at home.

A deductible combined with the basic account would also make us think about issues like which prescription drug best fulfills our needs. There are huge differences in the price of drugs, and as long as we believe they are free, we will always opt for the most expensive when, in fact, a generic drug may fulfill our needs. The next-generation health system must encourage our accountability and responsibility to bring efficiency and cost-effectiveness to the entire system.

3. *Catastrophe insurance*
After an individual has exhausted his or her basic health savings account and the deductible amount, catastrophe insurance comes into effect. This level of support is designed to cover costly emergency and disease care, and extensive and continuing costs for basic services. Catastrophe support would operate in a similar way as current health support, and the existing level of care would still be the minimum standard to which all Canadians are entitled but with different options.

The difference would be the way the insurance is implemented using the principles of health as the determining factors. For example, catastrophe care will have to be clearly defined. If it fails to meet the expectations of the patient, the system will have to find some way of allowing people to access what is most appropriate, even if the system cannot cover the costs.

Low-income Canadians and an HSA

As to which level of government could best resolve the issue, perhaps the community should be considered as part of the solution for the more personalized funding of these situations.

Canadians are very caring and supportive of their fellow citizens, and the thought of a deductible raises immediate concern for those who are unable to afford it. What will happen to the people who can't come up with the deductible? The most obvious solution is to include some form of alternative or graduated funding based on income or circumstances. This seems to make sense, but any compensating system must still encourage responsibility and accountability while not jeopardizing access to the basic levels of care. As to which level of government could best resolve the issue, perhaps the community should be considered as part of the solution for the more personalized funding of these situations.

Why Did the Romanow and Kirby Reports Reject HSAs?

The 2002 reports of both the Romanow Royal Commission and the Kirby Senate committee considered health savings accounts as alternatives to the existing funding model. Both came to the conclusion that the idea was impractical. The problem is that both studies were looking for ways to make the existing system work better, not alternatives to the system itself. Neither was looking for ways to empower the individual as the manager of his or her own personal health system. Both were politically motivated commissions and, at the time, it was political suicide even to consider reforming the health system.

There were three general problems with health savings accounts as an option for the existing system:

- Under the mandates of the studies, it was essential to have a funding mechanism to support our current system: being able to measure what we manage, and being able to offer exactly the same services to everyone. Health savings accounts encourage individuality, and work on the principle that the insurance is a benefit to help support the patient, not an all-inclusive funding system. This would be a major conflict.

- A funding mechanism such as an HSA that encourages us to be informed and responsible, to demand options and personally define quality would only create chaos for a system that is financially strained to the limits to provide the existing limited options for care.
- The HSA is dependent on empowered teams to provide all options and to manage the business aspects of direct payment, which is incompatible with the management model that the current Act supports.

Once again, if we change the way we look at things, the things we look at will change. If we begin to look at things from a patient and health perspective, then HSAs are one option that can fulfill all the criteria.

The People-Centred System and HSAs

In earlier chapters I have set out the criteria for a people-centred system. Here is a summary of how health savings accounts support each of the main criteria:

1. Each person is empowered to consider all health options, whether they are inside or outside the range of current possibilities. The HSA is able to recognize and reward all options.
2. We are designing a system that has the primary purpose of supporting the health of all Canadians. The HSA is consistent with a definition of health that is much broader than what the existing system is able to support.
3. We are searching for ways to make the system fit health, rather than compromising our health expectations to fit a system. The HSA puts health first.
4. The people-centred model demands choice and personally defining quality. The HSA encourages responsibility and accountability, which results in choices and a personal definition of quality for each of us.

5. The people-centred model demands that we accept reality, personally manage our own health system and use our strengths to overcome our weaknesses. The HSA encourages us to accept responsibility and our time, energy, social, financial and environmental realities.

6. A people-centred model means that the provider's rewards are outcome-based. The HSA empowers the patient, and creates an environment where the provider's and support group's success is based on fulfilling the needs of the patient.

7. The HSA responds to the need for a universal health safety net. It provides universal funding for a defined minimum level of care, with incentives for us to spend wisely and assume financial responsibility for our decisions.

8. The HSA supports rather than creates barriers to moving up the levels of the health care pyramid by allowing each of us to decide how we use our health care funding.

9. The HSA is consistent with the inverted management and legislative models of a people-centred health care system because it places responsibility on each patient to use the funding wisely.

10. The HSA system minimizes perverse incentives and limits abuse on the part of patients, providers, support groups and politicians.

11. The HSA (unlike other social-financing plans) does not force the patient to wait until the support group approves a procedure for financing. The funding is available, each of us is responsible for providing for our own needs, and a health coach helps determine the most appropriate treatment.

12. The HSA respects the fact that each of us is ultimately responsible for ourselves and that nearly all of us are capable of making decisions and choices about what is most appropriate for our needs.

13. New ideas about what basic services are delivered, who delivers them and where or when the services are delivered need not threaten the system or its financial viability. The HSA provides compensation that allows for a universally accepted level of care, with the individual free to choose a different level of care if it is more appropriate for his or her needs.

Canada is Ready for HSAs

The major problem with moving to a new model is knowing where and how to begin. With most health care funding proposals, it is all or nothing—either the whole system and philosophy changes or it fails. By contrast, Canada is quite ready for the transition to health savings accounts:

- We already have the system in place for catastrophe insurance.
- The HSA system can be introduced gradually, if necessary. There is no all-or-nothing requirement for how quickly we introduce the basic and deductible accounts. Depending on political will, Canada will be able to start small and grow as the need and the commitment grows. The amount of funding for the basic account or the amount of the deductible can be increased or decreased, whenever the funding is available. The minor services covered can also be readily adjusted.
- The HSA could first be introduced in smaller regions, if the public were hesitant to implement it nationally. This flexibility could also be very useful as the national economy fluctuates and the ability of the government to support health care changes. Regardless of what the universal health safety net can or cannot provide, if the individual and his or her provider are legally able to seek out options, the long-term success of the health safety net will be assured

The Next Step in our Action Plan

Because a health system is so complex, the sequence of events in a health reform plan is critical to a successful transition. As we saw in Chapter 5, designing a people-centred health Act is essential to the implementation of the other pieces of the puzzle. In discussions with many stakeholders and mentors, I have found unanimous agreement that a health savings account will only be effective if it is consistent with the rest of the system.

Once the *Canada Health and Wellness Act* is in place, it will be the driving force behind a transition to a funding system that supports the patient as the manager of his or her personal health system. Different funding mechanisms can work for different provider patient relationships, and a people-centred system must be flexible enough to incorporate whatever works for the individual or a particular support group. Nevertheless, developing the criteria for an appropriate funding framework is the vital second step in our action plan.

The third step is making sure that all stakeholders get the information they need for a people-centred health system, the focus of the next chapter.

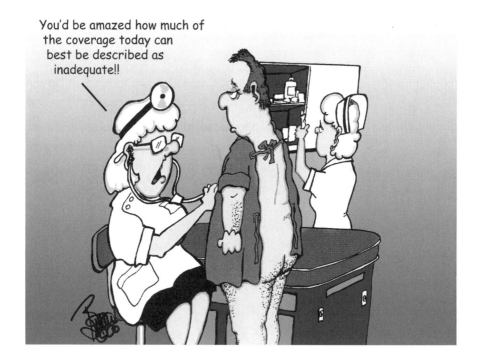

SUMMARY—CHAPTER 8

- introducing funding arrangements that support the definition and principles of health is critical to the success or failure of the people-centred system

- a people-centred system does not mean a person can buy access to care; it does mean that if an option is not covered or if a support group fails to provide a defined level of care, the patient can use whatever options are available to pursue his or her health goals

- Funding is vital to empowering the individual— the buck must stop with the patient if he or she is in control

- the combination of a health savings account, a deductible account and catastrophe insurance fulfills all the goals of a people-centred system

- all funding options can work, provided they are implemented without violating the principles of health

- there are creative ways to ensure the rights of all Canadians are protected regardless of income or social status

- health savings accounts are a form of funding that informs and empowers the client; it is not a good option in a system based on political or provider control

- Canada can implement health savings accounts as slowly or quickly as we wish

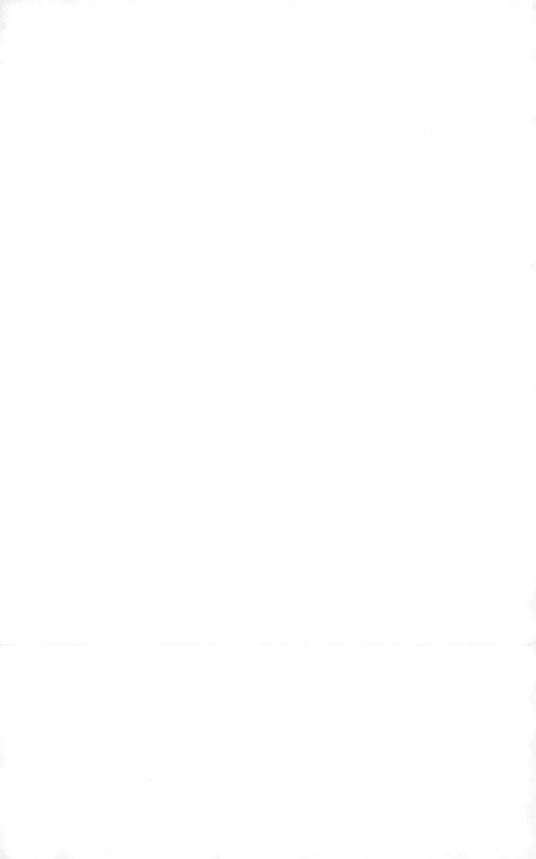

CHAPTER 9

Informing Canadians

Information is the key to understanding, designing and making a success of Canada's next-generation health system.

W E BELONG TO THE FIRST GENERATION of grassroots Canadians who can experience that knowledge is power. As Paul Hoffert suggests in *The New Client*, no individual, business or government can avoid the power of the information that people can acquire universally and instantly in our electronic age:

> Access to information, which used to be controlled by inter-mediary government and industry gatekeepers, is now available universally and instantly. An important consequence of this shift is the sense that instead of them (faceless government and business interests) keeping tabs on us (ordinary people), we are now watching them. The change is profound, derailing the expected Orwellian scenario in which Big Brother would control every aspect of our lives and replacing it with a scenario in which governments, businesses and suppliers of all sorts are accountable to the client.[41]

Health and health care are already the beneficiaries of this new power, and technology is what makes it possible.

To experience the rewards of a people-centred system, people must have access to information that can empower them. All that any system can aspire to do is make the information and options available and encourage and support each of us in every way possible as we make use of these benefits. The goal is not to force people to access

As people realize that personal responsibility and being informed are critical pieces on their personal health journey, the number of people using technology and demanding their providers do so will only increase.

information but to have a system that makes accessing and using the information an option. As people realize that personal responsibility and being informed are critical pieces on their personal health journey, the number of people using technology and demanding their providers do so will only increase.

This chapter outlines some of the ways that Canadians can get the information they need to be the managers of their personal health systems, the ways that information technology can help providers, and several information tools for governments.

Tools to Inform and Empower the People

There are many tools for informing and empowering individual Canadians. The exciting fact is that this is only the beginning. Thirty-two million stakeholders will find many other creative ways to share health information and experience the power that comes with it. I want to introduce some of the options that exist today or soon will be part of the information boom.

1. the human touch: one-on-one coaching
2. schools and education
3. the Internet
4. hotlines
5. information centres
6. patient advocacy groups
7. libraries and online resources
8. patient-centred portals
9. information technology for providers
10. electronic health records
11. technology-assisted diagnoses.

The human touch

Regardless of what technology is able to do, nothing will ever replace the power of one-on-one personal relationships with skilled communication and lis-

...nothing will ever replace the power of one-on-one personal relationships with skilled communication and listening.

tening. A personal coach is still the preferred way to process the information that technology can bring. The whole concept of a coach must be expanded to become the individual's primary information processing partner in health care.

Schools and education

School curricula must be part of the health care process. A child is never too young to begin his or her journey to wellness:

- The purpose of the health system is to support the health of Canadians, and the place to start is with national programs to inform and empower children before they become victims. It is easier to teach good health habits than it is to change them.
- Sharing health rights and responsibilities at a young age will go a long way to reducing dependency on the system.
- The education system can help young people to understand their personal responsibility for well-being, and that they will manage their health for over 99% of their lives.
- We can empower young people by challenging them to resolve health issues creatively and use the non-professional resources available. Health providers are there to support them, not rescue them.
- Teaching young people the six principles of health will be critical to developing a generation of personal health managers.

For a people-centred system to be successful, these ideas and many more must be part of the curricula, not only at all levels of primary and secondary education, but also in Canada's medical, nursing and alternative health training centres.

The Internet

The Internet will be a primary information centre for health care in the future. Governments can help, but it is the entrepreneurial spirit of the information technology industry that will lead the way in developing ideas for empowering individuals with the information they need to achieve their health goals.

To accomplish this we will need easily accessible websites that contain high quality information from reliable sources. Each of us also needs a trusted coach to help sort through the information and separate it from the misinformation.

Hotlines

To complement reliable websites, we need telephone hotlines for people who don't yet have access to the Internet in their homes or local public libraries, or who choose not to use it. An example is the Ontario government's *Telehealth* service (1-866-797-0000), which has registered nurses available 24/7 to answer questions and give advice on a large number of health issues.[42] The Canadian Society for Telehealth is the national body promoting reliable support networks.[43]

Information centres

Another possibility is a system of community information centres, augmented by kiosks (with Internet access) and mobile services, perhaps along the lines of Ontario's Early Years Centres. Funded by the provincial government and run by community groups, these centres provide information, programming and care tips for parents and caregivers of children in their formative years up to the age of six.[44] Similar information centres could be established on all aspects of health care for all ages.

Patient advocacy groups

There are many patient advocacy groups across the nation. Each has a particular interest, from access to prescription drugs and cancer treatment to heart disease. The interesting thing is that these groups have never united under a common vision. The Canadian Association for People-Centred Health (www. peoplecentredhealth.ca) has two goals. One is to be an advocate for a people-centred system. The second is to be the nucleus for all groups, professional organizations and corporations that are committed to informing, empowering and supporting the patient. Individually these groups can have some influence, but together they can become the driving force for the evolution of change in our health system.

Libraries and online resources

We must never forget the greatest user-friendly information resource in the country. Canada's 57,000 librarians—information management specialists—are possibly the greatest resource in the country for informing, empowering and supporting the health of the people.[45] Accessible in all communities and professionally trained to find information in all forms, they will play a major role in the evolving health model. A good deal of health information is available by subscription on commercial Internet sites, including those for medical journals and research reports. With the co-operation of Canada's public and educational libraries, much of this online information could be made available to anyone for a small fee or possibly as a community service.

Patient-centred portals

An example of the contributions that technology can make to the quality of life for people with health issues is the *My Care Source Patient Portal*, developed by Glen Kearns and Claudette Delenardo at Grand River Hospital in Kitchener, Ontario. Glen described the portal to me this way:

> Our health care system in Canada has lost the focus on the patient. All the processes, systems, buildings, applications, and equipment are designed around the providers. At Grand River Hospital that trend is starting to change and a new software application is an enabler of the change. *My Care Source* is a web based software application and portal currently available to all patients registered at the hospital's oncology service. The

hospital developed the application in partnership with McKesson Canada to accomplish three specific goals: empower the patient during the episode of care, include the patient as an active member of the care team, and change the model of care to become patient-centric (versus provider-centric). Today, over 180 patients are using the portal to take control of their destiny during some of the most difficult experiences in one's lifetime.

The patient portal allows patients to review their individual treatment plans week by week, service by service over the entire course of treatment, get specific educational materials about all aspects of their disease from recognized organizations, track and monitor their symptoms and side effects, build personal health profiles to form their own electronic health records, record their experiences in an online diary, get direct information about their care team members and other community support agencies, and be connected to the oncology program with a message centre directly in the portal. As one of the patients said, "Through the portal I can plan out the next two days and be prepared for the pending treatments."

Health care is the most complex industry on our planet— we should be using this type of technology to empower patients and put them at the centre of this dynamic industry. Grand River Hospital has taken initial steps to put patients at the centre and they continue to work with others to improve the health care experience for patients.

This is only one example of the patient centric research and programs that already exists. Creating a centre where all such programs can collaborate with a common vision to inform, empower and support will only enhance the quality of care and life for Canadians.

Information technology for providers

People-centred health practitioners must not only be exceptionally well-informed about their areas of practise, but they must also know how to assist their clients in getting appropriate information. Video and teleconferencing are already used for training providers. Information technology can help providers and patients to access information that will enhance the quality and timeliness of care and support the principles of people-centred health. As some of the available software is integrated into the system, it will be a major factor in future quality, timeliness, diagnosis and treatment-planning issues.

Telemedicine using various types of technology is now operating in many countries around the world. Also called e-health, it is proving particularly helpful in countries like Canada which have small settlements in remote areas without a full-time doctor or specialist. Diagnosis and even treatment of certain health problems are possible by using web cameras and video conferencing. A specialist in Ottawa or Toronto, for example, can rapidly bring a wide range of services to patients and providers in remote and underserved Northern communities by telephone, computer imaging over the Internet and teleconferencing, among others. Canadian governments are exploring further telehealth applications, as are the U.S. government's Office for the Advancement of Telehealth, state governments and the private sector.[46]

Electronic health records

Until recently, the technology was not available to gather and share the mass of information that will inform and empower individuals and allow them the option of being active participants in the management of their personal health. Major breakthroughs in the last few years, however, have resulted in software for handling comprehensive electronic health records. The evolution of technology creates a new set of issues:

- First, politicians can no longer blame technology for delaying the introduction of people-centric software. The real issue is whether our financially compromised health system wants to implement the technology and software that exists, and thus run the risk of having more informed patients putting even greater demands on the system.

- Another issue is getting providers and support groups to inte-grate this technology into their practises. One software com-pany candidly summarized the situation for me in these terms. We have three categories of providers: those who are friendly toward information technology and readily embrace the idea of technical support, a second group that is less enthusiastic but can see the benefits and is willing to go through a period of adjustment, and a third group that is waiting to retire. The problem is that too many of the more experienced leaders are in the third group, and they are the ones calling the shots.
- The final issue it getting the information to the public in a format that they can understand and use.

With the introduction of more sophisticated records such as MRIs and CT scans, the volume of information in our records has increased immensely, but several software companies such as XJ Partners in Toronto are currently developing systems for making all health records available securely online, including full diagnostic tests and records.[47] In Alberta, the province's Department of Health and Wellness has begun to set up the Alberta Electronic Health Records, a clinical health information network linking community physicians, hospitals, pharmacists and other authorized health care profession-als.[48] The network collects information about patients from across the province in one secure electronic view to make it easier for practitioners to assess and treat them.

The effect of this technology will be far-reaching. Accurate, legible records (unlike the average doctor's handwriting) are essential to moving to an effective, efficient, accountable and sustainable health system. Health care providers can invest as much as a quarter of their time maintaining handwritten records (a contributing factor in the shortage of doctors), and electronic records could free up a great deal of time in the average day for a general practitioner.

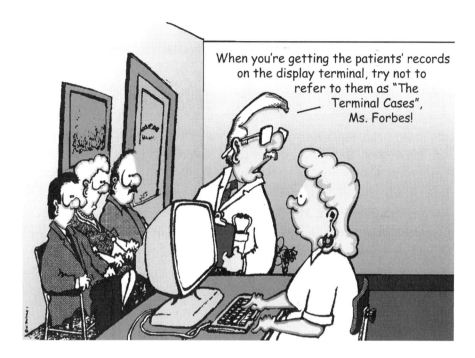

Technology-assisted diagnoses

A web search for computerized diagnostic centres in Canada will now bring up over 1,100 sites. The use of CT scans and MRIs has greatly enhanced the speed and accuracy of diagnosis and treatment planning. Moreover, computer technology can help providers access current information or a differential diagnosis on almost any health topic.[49] Using technology to assist in diagnoses can also help providers in the almost impossible task of keeping pace with research. An American researcher recently found from the medical records of participants in a survey that when there was a confirmed diagnosis and a recommended treatment, there was only a 55% chance of receiving the recommended treatment.[50]

But all the technology in the world is of no use if the health care system is not able to incorporate the technology rapidly and flexibly and cannot afford to offer the expanding number of options

Technology is only going to increase the demand for a system that allows what is possible rather than what a third party is willing or able to provide.

that are available. Technology is only going to increase the demand for a system that allows what is possible rather than what a third party is willing or able to provide.

The Need For Disclosing Information—Both Ways

I have become increasingly aware of the need for information disclosure between individuals and their providers—helping providers and patients to know one another. Individuals must never assume that their provider thinks as they do or that they share the same goals. It is essential that *both* providers and clients ask the questions that are necessary for them to have confidence in their health relationship. There are many types of doctors, and it is important for clients not to assume that all doctors are the same and ask some questions before they entrust their health to a particular health provider.

How doctors approach health care can be influenced by their political beliefs, their social consciences, where they were educated and the extent of their personal baggage. People have to remember that doctors are real people with values and needs and families and personal histories. Although interviewing a potential provider is rare, information technology could help us get the information we need to choose a doctor or provider with whom we feel comfortable. It is not that one doctor is right and another is wrong, but that every provider has a different style and it is in the best interests of our health that we connect with a provider who shares our values and approach to health.

Types of doctor–patient relationships

Generally speaking, we can identify four main types of doctor–patient relationships:

- the *guild* model: the doctor is all-knowing, and makes all the decisions because he or she knows what is best for the patient
- the *agent* model: the doctor only does what the patient asks of him or her
- the *commercial* model: the doctor uses market conditions and business principles to guide decisions. It is caveat emptor

(buyer beware) for the patient. In this scenario, fees are based on market pressure

- the *interactive* model: the provider, whether a doctor or coach, teaches the patient what he or she needs to know in order to make informed decisions. The provider answers the patient's questions and concerns, and they reach a common understanding on treatment.[51]

As you can imagine, a guild-model doctor practises medicine in a very different way from an interactive-model doctor. The guild doctor functions very well with the individual who says, "You know what's best, doc. I will do whatever you say." But the guild doctor has great difficulty with someone who has researched his or her health issue on the Internet, has many questions, and demands to have answers before accepting treatment. It is a waste of both the doctor's and the patient's time if they are not compatible in their approach to care.

The way to overcome this is disclosure. Many people are not comfortable interviewing a health professional. In fact there is such a shortage of providers that they fear confronting their providers with any questions because there are no options. Yet determining the kind of doctor–patient relationship we need is vital for long-term success in care. As providers' office websites become more common, this is the type of information that people should be able to have before they even make the initial phone call to a health provider's office.

Disclosing types of treatment

There are other types of questions you can ask your provider. For instance, a common misconception is that the doctor is treating the problem rather than the symptom of the problem. It is important that we ask our provider or coach about this and discuss alternatives. In any treatment, we should ask whether we are being treated for the symptom or for the cause of the symptoms. If the provider is treating the symptom, then it is logical for us to ask about the cause and what can we do to eliminate the cause or causes.

Let me illustrate with an example. Catherine goes to a doctor with a persistent headache. The doctor prescribes a muscle relaxant or painkiller. Catherine has every right to ask whether the prescription will treat the cause or the symptom. Pain is a symptom and we want to get rid of it as quickly as possible, but it will almost always recur if we only treat the symptom. If you treat the cause, then eliminating the symptoms may take longer, but the goal is to prevent the recurrence of symptoms. The issue for a system that is financially compromised and struggling with a perceived shortage of providers is that it is much more time-consuming and costly to diagnose and treat causes than it is to treat symptoms. Governments want to reduce waiting lists and minimize costs. The more people who are seen by the fewer number of providers, the greater the chance of fulfilling both these objectives. The result is that we have a health system that is geared to treating symptoms. Muscle relaxants, pain medication and antidepressants are too often used as a quick fix so that the provider can get to the next patient. By asking our providers to tell us whether they are treating symptoms or causes, each of us can begin a very different doctor–patient relationship and move from treating illness to sup-porting health and gaining control of our health issues.

In my discussions with Dr. Bruce Squires, a past editor of the *Canadian Medical Association Journal* and a member of several inter-national committees of the World Association of Medical Editors, he shared with me the six questions he believes people should ask their providers about health issues:

1. What's the diagnosis? How certain are you?
2. What are my options (including doing nothing)?
3. What are the benefits of each option?
4. What are the risks of each?
5. Once I have chosen an option, who is the best person to do the treatment? What is his or her record of success and failure?
6. What is the prognosis?

Take these along as a starting point for discussions about your next health issue. You might be pleasantly surprised how the conversation with a provider can change when you change the way you look at things.

Information Tools For Governments

The federal, provincial and territorial governments can inform, empower and support the people by providing information in many ways. Perhaps the most important first step will be the initial public discussions and debate about designing a people-centred health system, and developing a *Canada Health and Wellness Act* that supports this vision. But governments' educational mission does not stop there. They could:

- set up *national websites*: just as the Canadian Association for People-Centred Health and many other voluntary associations will make patient advocacy a focus of their websites, so too can governments expand their sites to include far more detailed and linked health information than they currently provide
- create *cross-Canada information repositories*: available to everyone, regional and local repositories of health care information could be supplemented by Internet access points in libraries, schools and recreation and community centres
- continue developing *the information highway*: governments could assist the private sector in expanding fibre-optic cable and satellite access to the Internet for all Canadians, especially in remote and underserved areas
- encourage and reward communication by health provider teams: governments could offer explicit incentives in the *Canada Health and Wellness Act*, and
- promote *well-being*: all governments could promote health and health care in ways that can be demonstrated to have an measurable effect, not by feel-good or self-congratulatory advertising.

Information, in a word, is the key to understanding, designing and making a success of Canada's next-generation health system. Now let's see how it will work in practise.

SUMMARY—CHAPTER 9

- information is the key to understanding, designing and making a success of Canada's next-generation health system
- changing the way we look at things is essential to the evolution of health care: developing a positive, entrepreneurial attitude where all things are possible is the first step
- there are at least 11 ways to access and share information that will enable the people-centred health system to thrive
- disclosing information about all aspects of a health relationship is vital
- ask your health care provider six questions
- governments should inform the people in five ways

CHAPTER 10

How a People-Centred Model Works

A visit to a people-centred doctor's office is built on trusting relationships.

THIS BOOK'S people-centred model of health care for Canadians is based on my 30 years' experience in dentistry, founded on a team approach to empowering clients. It sounds great in theory, but does it work? In this chapter I answer some frequently asked questions, and suggest what might happen during a typical visit to the doctor.

1. Will I Be Able to Get The Same Level of Care As I Have Now?

Yes. There is nothing in people-centred reform that will prevent you from getting the existing level of care, which will represent the minimum level of care that all Canadians are entitled to. Moreover, you would no longer be limited in the optimum level of care you could access, or the quality of care a provider could offer, if the system is unable or unwilling to offer it.

2. What Level of Support Can I Expect?

The minimum level of support will be the very best that society is able and willing to provide through the limited resources of the tax system. There is no such thing as a universal level of support that can be all things to all people.

When I first started discussing a people-centred system, I would ask the audience to pretend that there was a major catastrophe. By some twist of fate you were on a committee to create a health support system for the country. What would you do? The premise was that society wanted to provide a universal level of support to ensure that all people could have access to a defined level of care. If we were part of such a committee, each of us would have to answer two basic questions: What support am I willing to offer the other people in the room? and What would I expect the other people in the room to do for me?

It seems ludicrous that people expect society to provide support for all people, if we were not willing to make the same sacrifice for someone we know or love. It is unrealistic to expect others to give up everything to ensure that participants would have unlimited, unconditional support, regardless of what they do or how they manage their health, so why do people expect a government to? The real issue is how much and what form of support society should provide. As people consider the implications, they quickly become aware that there have to be limits to what any support group can offer, and these limits must be clearly defined.

3. Who Will Manage The System?

An independent, non-political health care commission is the final level of support in the people-centred management model. This commission is like the highest court in the judicial system and is responsible for enforcing the *Canada Health and Wellness Act*. Although the Act is brought in by the federal government and administered provincially, and only the government has the right to change it, management will no longer be a political football bounced around by public opinion polls.

4. Will My Rights Be Protected?

Yes, better than they ever have been until now:

- First, information and records will be readily available, services will be clearly defined and governments will be accountable to the commission and to the people for their promises.

- Second, you can no longer be held hostage to a government that does not deliver on its promises. If the government fails to deliver, it will be the right of all people to pursue options.
- Third, the right to informed consent will finally be entrenched in the system.
- Finally, the principles of health will be enforced by the commission for all aspects of the health system.

5. What Will It Be Like When I Visit My Doctor?

Quite different from what you may be used to now. In the first place, you'll most likely notice that the staff members have somewhat different titles and responsibilities. A single-practitioner office, for example, might have two receptionists, two case managers (preferably nurses), two nurse practitioners and the general practitioner. The whole team would be co-ordinated by an office manager. This team of eight people with an integrated software program and technical support could effectively and efficiently manage a large number of clients in a very caring, people-centred way.

A common complaint I hear about the current system is that "I walk out feeling like I don't know what happened or whether anyone really listened or cared." In the patient-centred system, the initial examination is the first critical step. Properly done, a sound patient–provider relationship is launched.

The initial examination is not performed by a doctor alone. To be successful, it requires a team approach by a health care team who understand one another's strengths and skills. They work together to find the most effective way of helping you to define your personal health and health care goals.

After the initial examination, let's say that you have a chronic headache and want an appointment. You phone the receptionist, who clarifies your needs and arranges an appointment as soon as possible with your personal coach (one of the case managers or nurse practitioners determined at your initial examination). When you arrive, the coach records the details of your medical problem. The doctor then comes in, reviews what the coach has learned, examines you, and presents you with your options. Unless your headache is a life-threatening problem, the decision on what you should do is up to you (and your coach, if you wish). Once you have determined which option you wish to pursue, the coach explains the costs and together you explore ways to achieve your goals. If at any time there is a need for clarification from the doctor, the coach (as your advocate) will seek clarification immediately and discuss it with you.

A people-centred office experience is built around trusting relationships. By introducing the option for the patient to have a coach or client co-ordinator other than the doctor, all things become possible. With the shortage of physicians it is impossible for a doctor to invest this kind of time in relationships, but if most patient visits can be coached or managed by someone other than the doctor, and if there is a system in place that allows people other than the doctor to fulfill this role and be rewarded (either by the system or personally), then we have enhanced the quality of care and reduced the strain on the doctor.

Detailed Example of a Patient-centred Examination

This example highlights five aspects of a typical client examination, with *comments in italics*. The example does not involve an emergency, which would follow different procedures. The participants are:

- Jane, the patient
- Paula, the receptionist
- Pam, the coach, and
- Dr. Well, the physician.
- Jane recently turned 50 and has not seen a doctor for six years. She does not have any serious problems, but wants to get back on track to feeling better.

The phone interview

Jane phones for an examination. Paula, the receptionist, completes a screening interview to assess Jane's needs and set up an examination. She explains that there are several examination options. *Even at the initial phone call Jane has choices. Not all patients are the same, so why would one exam procedure fit everyone? Emergencies are dealt with immediately and are very focused, but for someone such as Jane, Paula would suggest a comprehensive examination.* Paula does not go into great detail, but attempts to find out enough about Jane's personal history and her health concerns so that she can arrange an examination process that meets her expectations. *Paula is also trying to determine who might be the most appropriate team member to be the initial client co-ordinator or coach.* She quotes a fee range based on the needs that emerged in the telephone call.

The patient interview

On the day of the examination, Pam, a coach, greets Jane and escorts her to a consultation room for a personal interview. *The coach, also called a client co-ordinator, could be a nurse practitioner, a nurse or a trained greeter, but rarely the doctor.* They get to know one another and share personal and health-related facts. It is at this time that they design a personally relevant examination together. *Typically this takes 20–30 minutes for a trained team member, and is critical to the long-term provider–patient relationship. During this time the coach invites the patient to share past and present concerns and experiences, so that the coach can appreciate the patient as a real person. The patient senses genuine concern and feels she has been listened to: the first step in establishing a trusting relationship.*

The examination

Pam calls in Dr. Well, introduces Jane and brings the doctor up to date on their conversation so far. *This is preferably done in a consultation room, not the examination room, and in front of the patient, for two reasons: to reassure Jane that the coach was listening and to give Jane a chance to hear and confirm her history and concerns.* Dr. Well then asks pertinent questions and goes into detail about any concerns Jane has about her health history. He explains that the purpose of the examination is to gather as much information about Jane's health as possible, share the information with her, discuss options and make recommendations for future care.

Dr. Well, Pam and Jane move to an examination room and together they complete the examination. *As well as the usual medical procedures, the physical examination involves many listening and communication skills. For example, the doctor dictates all information aloud for the coach to record so that the patient is aware of everything.* At the end of the physical examination, Dr. Well asks Jane what she thinks of the information she heard. *This is a crucial step because it allows the doctor and the coach to focus on what is important and relevant to the patient's needs and values. Often the patient has a primary concern that is different from the doctor's, but as long as it is not an emergency the patient is always right. This may also be the first time that the patient has been invited to participate directly, conveying the idea that her opinion matters. It also begins to reinforce the concept that she has ownership of and responsibility for her own health.*

Treatment consultation

Dr. Well summarizes all the findings and outlines to Jane and the coach the options for proceeding. At this time, the options for treatment may or may not be clearly defined, and there may be several ways to proceed in gathering more information. *The important thing is that there are always options and the patient is invited to share in the decisions about where to go next.* Depending on the situation and Jane's decisions, Dr. Well answers any questions and explains that Pam will go through things in detail. The doctor leaves, and Jane and her coach review the options and decide how to proceed. If at any time the doctor's opinion is needed, Pam will call in Dr. Well. *The patient-centred examination usually takes 30 to 40 minutes for the doctor and 1 to 2 hours for the coach. Serious health problems may require the doctor to be present at all times, but for most health concerns the doctor and coach discuss the options, and the coach and patient discuss the how, when, where, and why of treatment. By the time the exam is completed, typically the patient and her coach—and, we hope, the doctor—have made the first steps to establishing a trusting relationship. The patient has developed confidence that she can share information and that her coach will act in her best interests.* When Jane is comfortable that she has all the information she needs, she makes an appointment with Paula for treatment, the next step of her health journey.

Financial arrangements

For this first examination, Paula presents Jane with the bill for the fee they agreed on, Jane approves it and authorizes payment from her health savings account. Now it is up to Jane and her coach or possibly even a financial co-ordinator to explore ways to achieve her goals, and to find other support groups to assist in areas where her resources or benefits are inadequate.

Financing and treatment options

More generally, in the example of Jane and her health care team it is essential to understand that none of the procedures or options was determined by what a third-party insurance company or a government health program covers. The options are determined by the findings of the clinical examination. The treatment plan is established by what the patient and the doctor or coach agree is the best way to fulfill the health needs of the patient. Financial arrangements then become a process of canvassing what benefits are available to the patient, and exploring ways by which they can achieve their health goals. Whether funding is through a health savings account, a fee-for-service arrangement or a payment-per-person (capitation) scheme, the examination procedure, the options available and the treatment-plan decisions of the patient should be the same. Otherwise the insurance company is dictating treatment, and in my view it is unethical to have a third party dictate the relationship between a patient and his or her provider.

In Jane's case, the steps in her initial examination may seem somewhat lengthy. But each step of the examination is important if the goal is to be a well-informed and empowered patient. In the examination the patient usually needs time to talk, to be listened to and to get clarification. It makes sense that someone who has the time and the listening and communication skills should be present throughout, and that the doctor only does what he or she must legally do: to make a diagnosis and define treatment options. Patients can choose the more expensive option of having their doctors undertake all steps of the complete examination, but if their financial support program does not cover it, they always have the option of doing only what is covered. If they are paying through their personal health savings accounts or out of their own pockets, there is a great incentive to understand the options and choose what is the most effective, efficient and financially acceptable alternatives.

Jane has the responsibility for choosing which option is most appropriate at various times during the process, from the first phone call to the completion of the exam and final consultation. She feels valued and listened to, and appreciates that her input is essential. She has started a relationship based on trust, and probably feels very comfortable with a doctor who is open and willing to trust his team members.

Perhaps our hypothetical patient Jane—who was given a copy of the people-centred report card by her coach, Pam—may not feel the need to assess her initial examination. This was her first experience with people-centred health care, after all, and her overwhelming impression on all levels was that it was substantially better than the old system. In fact, she probably wouldn't have experienced any equivalent under the former system. Her examination under a people-centred system is not a requirement; it is an option, and it should be an alternative.

The problem is that the current system cannot afford this kind of an examination universally, and the government cannot measure and manage this quality of care. Only the patient can assess whether it is appropriate and of value, and only then if she is the manager of her own health system. Once this has really sunk in, Jane will be quite ready to assess her treatment.

SUMMARY—CHAPTER 10

- people will be able to access the same level of care as they do now

- support will continue to be the very best that society is willing and able to provide; the difference is that the government will be held much more accountable for its promises

- all stakeholders (including the government) will be accountable to a non-partisan health care commission, which in turn is accountable to the *Canada Health and Wellness Act* setting out the definitions and principles of a people-centred health model

- the examination procedure is the ultimate test of the system

CHAPTER 11

The Ticket for
Our Journey to Wellness

The challenge for society is not to create barriers so that all people are treated equally, but to support all people equally so we can all have the opportunity to pursue our highest potentials. The vision and leadership for health care reform can come only from the people.

O N A FAMILY NEW YEAR'S VACATION this year I was reflecting on how to conclude this introduction to our journey to wellness. Just a few days earlier, on 26 December 2004, a vast tsunami had hit Southeast Asia and the news broadcasts were focused on the terrible tragedy. An event like this reminds us once again of our insignificance in the big picture, the overwhelming power of nature and the inability of any man made system to overcome its power. The number of people dead and missing was enormous, and there was little or nothing that money, power or research could do for these people.

The pictures of lives and families being destroyed and interviews with the survivors motivated people in all nations to support one of the largest humanitarian aid programs the world has ever seen, and yet it seems so insignificant compared with the personal loss for which no amount of material giving could compensate.

Yet tsunami-like events sweep across North America every year and we choose to ignore them. They take the lives of hundreds of thousands of people, and we cannot buy, give or legislate anything that will stop the devastating tidal waves caused by alcohol, illegal drugs, smoking, diabetes and obesity, among others. The solution lies within each of us, and society must stop trying to be the saviour and recognize that its role is to support. Rescuing and saving only makes us more dependent victims. We must look to ourselves if we want to stop this death and destruction. The essential challenge is ours to undertake, not society's.

Canadians are among the luckiest people in the world to have a society that is committed to giving all people access to a basic level of health care. But this is only the beginning, and it is time to build on what Tommy Douglas and many others have given us. To continue our collective journey to wellness, individuals must accept responsibility for what and who we are, learn about our options, define what quality of life we want, make choices, and understand that all any of us can do is the best with what we have to work with.

Perhaps the greatest threat to our Canadian way of life is our obsession with illness care and our refusal to accept the limitations of what money can do to fulfill this obsession. Attempting to buy health by treating illness is beginning to have an overwhelming effect on all social programs. We must accept that if Canadians were to abandon all other social programs and invest every penny of tax revenues into the services we now cover in our universal illness-care system, everyone will eventually get sick and die.

The reality is that there is no universal solution to treating illness or supporting health, because both are ultimately determined by what individuals do for themselves, not what others do for them. We must accept this fact, define the limits of what our publicly funded health safety net is expected to do to support the health of the people, and live within our means.

What makes this an even greater threat is that the decisions are being left in the hands of politicians, who have not gone through the process of developing a vision for health, and whose primary goal is to get elected. As a senior advisor to Ontario's Minister of Health told me, "the vision and leadership for health care reform can come only from the people."

As a society we must start to inform, empower and support the people. Each of us is mortal. Most Canadians die sooner because of what they will not do for themselves, rather than what others are not willing to do for them.

The challenge for society is not to create barriers so that all people are treated equally, but to support all people equally so they can all have the opportunity to pursue their highest potentials. There is nothing we as a society can do to make people pursue their highest potential.

The challenge for each of us to become all we are capable of is personal, and the answer does not lie with a political party, a health provider or new technology. The ticket for our journey to wellness is inside each one of us!

CHAPTER 12

A Call to Action!

Only you can fix Canada's health care crisis, but what can you do?

MOST CANADIANS ARE SURPRISED to find that our health system is really not centred around the people it is meant to support. The quality of our lives and in many situations life and death are, dependent on answering the questions and implementing policies that will make a difference. We have only just begun the journey.

The evolution of our system will only occur when the people demand it. This book is one way to share what I have learned and challenge each of you to be part of the solution. If there are problems with the system then the people must have the courage to ask the questions and either find answers or demand that those who claim to be leaders find the answers.

As my research continued and public interest grew in designing a health system around the people, it became clear that there must be something after this book is published that enables people to continue their personal journey and to give feedback. The Canadian Associatin for People-Centred Health (CAPCH) is not for profit and is meant to be your association. It will allow the average Canadian to provide input or make a contribution. Whether it is by becoming a member, getting regular updates, providing financial support or making a contribution through time and energy, the choice is yours.

The exciting part is that we can all be part of the creation of a health support network that is designed by the people and for the people.

There are two ways to make a difference:

1. *Make a difference personally:*

- Use the six principles of health – outlined in Chapter 3 — to evaluate your personal journey. Discover your individuality, accept ownership and responsibility for your well-being, seek information, seek out options and make choices, define the quality that meets your needs and most importantly accept reality and the fact that all any of us can hope for is to be all we are capable of.
- Join the Canadian Association for People-Centred Health and use the resources and links it offers to pursue your personal journey to wellness and to help others to do the same.

2. *Make a difference in the future of our health system:*

- Be a leader or at least be active in health issues and policies in your community. Encourage your local health leaders and providers to use the six principles of health to evaluate their support or care.
- We need a strong, united voice to make politicians sit up and listen. If you believe that Canadians should have the option to become all they are capable of, with a personally defined balance of mental, physical, spiritual and emotional well-being, then why not do your part to support the evolution of our system? Support the CAPCH
- Help us develop links to other groups and persons who share this patient-first approach. The CAPCH is meant to be a resource to connect all people-centred organizations. Visit our website at **www.peoplecentredhealth.ca** and get the most recent information about our ongoing research and teaching and also to connect with other people-centred organizations.
- Give us feedback on this book. Be a critic and share your ideas that would improve this vision. Share it with others and encourage them to read and learn about the system.

Contacting the Canadian Association for People-Centred Health

website: **www.peoplecentredhealth.ca**

mail: CAPCH

P.O.Box 309

Arnprior, Ontario

K7S-3H6

ENDNOTES

Introduction

1. *The Power of Intention: Learning to Co-Create Your World Your Way* (Carlsbad, California: Hay House, 2004), ch. 15.

CHAPTER 1

2. *Ottawa Citizen*, 7 May 2004, pp. 1, 6, 7, reporting on Nadeem Esmail, Michael Walker and Sabrina Yeudall, *How Good Is Canadian Health Care? 2004 Report* (Fraser Institute Critical Issues Bulletin 2004; Vancouver, May 2004).

3. The most recent version of the Act is available on the Health Canada Web site: **http://www.hc-sc.gc.ca/medicare/Canada%20Health%20Act.htm** [cited 9 May 2005].

4. Kelly Egan, "Vaughan Glover outwits our neighbour's sharpest minds to win $10,000 contest", *Ottawa Citizen*, 3 November 2003.

5. Mohammed Adam, "Doctors call drug deal with government a 'bribe'", *National Post*, 2 October 2004; Coalition of Family Physicians (Toronto), bulletins on "The Art of the Deal", 1 (19 October 2004) through 5 and 6 (8 November 2004), available at **www.cofp.com** [cited 13 May 2005]; Janice Tibbets, "Medicare goes on trial at Supreme Court", *National Post*, 7 June 2004.

6. Long Range Health Planning Branch, Department of Health and Welfare, *A New Perspective on the Health of Canadians: A Working Document* (Ottawa, 1974). The Hon. Marc Lalonde was Minister of Health and Welfare at the time; the document was a Green Paper: that is, a planning paper that does not necessarily reflect the government's policy intentions.

7. See Colleen M. Flood and Tom Archibald, "The Illegality of Private Health Care in Canada", *Canadian Medical Association Journal*, vol. 164 (2001), 825–830.

8. Patti Edgar, "Top cancer specialist heads to U.S.", *Ottawa Citizen*, 6 November 2002, p. B1.

9. Canadian Institute for Health Information, "Health Care Spending to Reach $130 Billion This Year; per capita Spending to Hit $4,000", 8 December 2004, Table A.2.1 ("Total Health Expenditure by Source of Finance, Canada, 1975 to 2004—Current Dollars"), a news release announcing the publication of *National Health Expenditure Trends, 1975–2004* at **http://secure.cihi.ca/cihiweb/dispPage. jsp?cw_page=media_08dec2004_e** [cited 9 May 2005]. The amounts for 2004 are preliminary.

10. Paule Boothe and Mary Carson, *What Happened to Health-Care Reform?* (C.D. Howe Institute Commentary no. 193; Toronto, December 2003), p. 16.

11. Canadian Institute for Health Information, op. cit., Table B.1.2 ,"Total Health Expenditure, by Province/Territory and Canada, 1975 to 2004—Current Dollars (Per Capita). The amounts for 2004 are preliminary.

12. As of 31 March 2003 (the latest data available), the consolidated net debt of the federal, provincial, territorial and local governments was $794.5 billion (Statistics Canada, *The Daily,* 25 April 2005). Assuming an average interest rate of 4.91% (the rate reported by the federal Department of Finance for 2003–2004 in its *Debt Management Report 2003–2004* at **http://www.fin.gc.ca/dtman/2003-2004/dmt04_2e.html** [cited 9 May 2005]) and a population of 31,747,670 (for 1 October 2003: *Statistics Canada, The Daily*, 24 March 2005), the interest costs would have been approximately $1,228.70 for each resident of Canada.

13. *Shaping Ontario's Physician Workforce: Building Ontario's Capacity to Plan, Educate, Recruit and Retain Physicians to Meet Health Needs: Report of the Expert Panel on Health Professional Human Resources* (Toronto: Ministry of Health and Long-Term Care, 2001), p. 9.

14. *How Good Is Canadian Health Care?*, p. 5.

15. "[F]unding constraints can mean that in some cases the [CT and MRI] equipment is only used 40 hours a week (sitting idle 16 hours a day and all weekend)": Medical Imaging Technology Roadmap Steering Committee, *Medical Imaging Discussion Paper* (Ottawa: ORTECH for Industry Canada, 1999), s. 4.5.10 at **strategis.ic.gc.ca/epic/internet/inmitr-crtim.nsf/en/h_hm01519e.html** [cited 13 May 2005].

16. Canadian Institute for Health Information, *RNDB: Registered Nurses Database: Workforce Trends of Registered Nurses in Canada, 2003* (Ottawa: CIHI, 2004), accompanying CD-ROM, data table E.RN.1.

17. Standing Senate Committee on Social Affairs, Science and Technology, *The Health of Canadians: The Federal Role—Final Report.* Vol. 6: *Recommendations for Reform* (Hon. Michael J.L. Kirby, Chair; Ottawa: The Senate, 2002); Commission on the Future of Health Care in Canada, *Building on Values: The Future of Health Care in Canada—Final Report* (Hon. Roy J. Romanow, Commissioner; Ottawa: The Commission, 2002).

18. "Summary of Median Wait Times for Services, by Type of Procedure and Local Health Integration Network, in Ontario, 2003/04" in J.V. Tu et al., *Access to Health Services in Ontario: ICES Atlas* (Toronto: Institute for Clinical Evaluative Services, 2005).

19. *Code Blue: Reviving Canada's Health Care System* (Toronto: ECW Press, 1999), pp. 142–145. Used with permission.

20. "Revisiting the *Canada Health Act* (1984): What are the Impediments to Change?", Institute on Public Policy, 30th Anniversary Conference, Ottawa, 20 February 2002.

21. Michael Rachlis and Carol Kushner, *Second Opinion: What's Wrong with Canada's Health Care System and How to Fix It* (Toronto: Collins, 1989), p. 7.

CHAPTER 2

22. Abraham Maslow, *Motivation and Personality* (2nd ed.; New York: Harper and Row, 1970).

23. Maslow, pp. xii, 57, 46.

24. Colossians 4:14; Luke 6:38.

25. "Constitution of the World Health Organization" in *World Health Organization: Basic texts* (44th ed.; Geneva: WHO, 2004) at **http://policy.who. int/cgi-bin/om_isapi.dll?hitsperheading=on&infobase=basicdoc&jump= Constitution&softpage=Document42#JUMPDEST_Constitution** [cited 9 May 2005].

26. WHO Regional Office for Europe, *Policy Statements* at **http://www.euro. who.int/AboutWHO/Policy/20010827_2** [cited 9 May 2005].

CHAPTER 3

27. Canadian Medical Association, "Number of Physicians by Province/Territory and Specialty, Canada, 2005" at **www.cma.ca/multimedia/CMA/ Content_Images/Inside_cma/Statistics/dem-number1.pdf** [cited 9 May 2005].

28. Canadian Institute for Health Information, "RN Workforce by Province/ Territory of Registration, Canada, 1999–2003" (241,342 for 2003), "LPN Workforce by Province/Territory of Registration/Licensure, Canada, 2002–2003" (63,138 for 2003), and "RPN Workforce by Province of Registration, Canada, 2003–2003" (5,107 for 2003), for a total of 309,587, at **http://secure.cihi.ca/cihiweb/dispPage. jsp?cw_page=statistics_a_z_e#D** [cited 9 May 2005].

29. "In studies of patient behaviour, only about half of patients who leave a physician's office with a prescription take the drug as directed": *Merck Manual of Diagnosis and Therapy*, s. 22, ch. 301 at **www.merck.com/mrkshared/mmanual/ section22/chapter301/301d.jsp** [cited 9 May 2005]; "research has proven that non-compliance is a serious medical issue. It is a major medical problem that may lead to death and elevated costs, both for patients and providers: Albert J. Wertheimer, "Medication Compliance Research: Still So Far to Go", *Journal of Applied Research in Clinical and Experimental Therapeutics*, III.3 (Summer 2003) at **jrnlapplied research.com/articles/Vol3Iss3/Wertheimer.htm** [cited 9 May 2005].

30. "More than half of all Americans with chronic diseases don't follow their physician's medication and lifestyle guidance": American Heart Association, "Statistics on Lifestyle Compliance" at **www.americanheart.org/presenter. jhtml? identifier = 107** [cited 9 May 2005].

31. *The New Client: How Customers Shape Business in the Information Age* (Toronto: Viking, 2002), p. 7.

32. For example, see *The Relationship between the Socioeconomic Status and Health of the Elderly* (RAND Research Bulletin RB-5020; Santa Monica, California: RAND Corporation, 1998) and Rebecca A. Clay, "Wealth Secures Health", *Monitor on Psychology* III.2 (October 2001).

33. *Man's Search for Meaning: An Introduction to Logotherapy* (Boston: Beacon, 1963), a revised version of the translation *From Death-Camp to Existentialism: A Psychiatrist's Path to a New Therapy* (Boston: Beacon, 1959).

34. $794.5 billion as at 31 March 2003, the most recent figure: see note 12 to chapter 1 above. The federal debt was $526.5 billion ($56.5 billion higher than it was 10 years earlier) and the debt of the provinces, territories and local governments was $268 billion.

CHAPTER 4

35. Rachlis and Kushner, *Second Opinion*, p. 55.

36. Health Services Restructuring Commission, *Primary Health Care Strategy* (Toronto: The Commission, November 1999), p. 16.

CHAPTER 6

37. The winning bid for the most recent five-year contract was $449,000,000: Glen McGregor, "Panel to rule soon on Calian medical deal with Forces", *Ottawa Citizen*, 10 May 2005, p. A3.

CHAPTER 7

38. College of Family Physicians of Canada, Canadian Medical Association and Royal College of Physicians and Surgeons of Canada, *Initial Data Release of the 2004 National Physician Survey* (Ottawa: CFPC, CMA and RCPSC, October 2004), p. 1.

39. Health Services Restructuring Commission, *Primary Health Care Strategy*, p. 16.

CHAPTER 8

40. *How Good Is Canadian Health Care? 2004 Report*, p. 3.

CHAPTER 9

41. *The New Client*, p. 9.

42. For further information, see the *Telehealth* Web site at **www.health.gov.on.ca/ english/public/program/telehealth/telehealth_mn.html** [cited 12 May 2005].

43. The Web site of the Canadian Society for Telehealth is available at **www.cst-sct. org/index.php**.

44. Information on Ontario's Early Years Centres appears on the centres' Web site: **http://www.ontarioearlyyears.ca/oeyc/en/home.htm**.

45. Canada has two main associations of librarians, each with a Web site: the Canadian Library Association **www.cla.ca** and L'Association des bibliothécaires du Québec **www.abqla.qc.ca**.

46. See *Rural Health/Telehealth* (Synthesis ser.; Ottawa: Health Canada, 2002), available on Health Canada's Health Transition Fund Web site at **http://www.hc-sc.gc.ca/htf-fass/english/** [cited 12 May 2005].

47. The company's Web site address is **www.xjpartners.com**.

48. The province's *Alberta Wellnet* Web site includes links to information about the Electronic Health Records network at **www.albertawellnet.org**.

49. See, for example, Monique Frize at al., "Clinical Decision-Support Systems for Intensive Care Units Using Artificial Neural Networks", *Medical Engineering and Physics*, vol. 23, no. 3 (April 2001), pp. 217–225 and other publications a **www.sce. carleton.ca/faculty/frize/MIRG_2001/publications.html** [cited 12 May 2005].

50. Elizabeth McGlynn et al., "The Quality of Health Care Delivered to Adults in the United States", *New England Journal of Medicine*, vol. 348 (2003), pp. 2635–2645.

51. Adapted from Dr. Barry Schwartz, "Dental Ethics: A Review of Current Literature", *Ontario Dentist* (December 2001).